D1445878

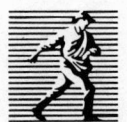

GOOD NEWS ABOUT HIGH BLOOD PRESSURE

Everything You Need to Know
to Take Control of Hypertension
—And Your Life

THOMAS PICKERING, M.D.

SIMON & SCHUSTER
New York • London • Toronto • Sydney • Tokyo • Singapore

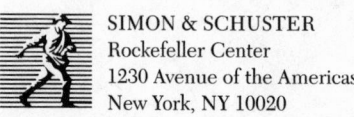

SIMON & SCHUSTER
Rockefeller Center
1230 Avenue of the Americas
New York, NY 10020

Copyright © 1996 by Thomas G. Pickering, M.D.
All rights reserved,
including the right of reproduction
in whole or in part in any form.
SIMON & SCHUSTER and colophon are registered trademarks
of Simon & Schuster Inc.
Designed by Irving Perkins Associates
Manufactured in the United States of America
10 9 8 7 6 5 4 3 2 1
Library of Congress Cataloging-in-Publication Data
Pickering. Thomas G.
Good news about high blood pressure : everything you need to know
to take control of hypertension—and your life / Thomas Pickering.
p.   cm.
Includes bibliographical references and index.
1. Hypertension—Popular works.   I. Title.
RC685.H8P513   1996
616.1'32—dc20   95-45136
CIP

ISBN 0-684-81396-3

ACKNOWLEDGMENTS

I would like to acknowledge the contributions that my patients have made, wittingly or unwittingly, to the writing of this book. In particular, Marie Tenebruso has painstakingly read and criticized the entire manuscript, and I am indebted to her for this. I also thank my secretary, Anna Christian, for her unflagging support, and my wife, Janet, for her help with the manuscript. Finally, I should also recognize the enthusiastic support of my agent, Perry Knowlton of Curtis Brown, and Fred Hills from Simon & Schuster.

To my patients, from whom I have learned so much.

CONTENTS

PREFACE

High blood pressure, or hypertension as it is medically called, affects about 50 million people in the United States. In the vast majority it produces no symptoms, but is important because, if unchecked, it can result in heart disease and strokes, which are the leading causes of death and disability. A recent government survey showed that while 65 percent of people with high blood pressure were aware of their condition, only 49 percent were being treated for it, and a mere 21 percent had their blood pressure adequately controlled.

For most people with hypertension it is a lifelong condition whose exact cause is unknown, although both heredity and the environment are thought to play a part. The good news is that there is a lot you can do to keep it in check and to prevent its consequences. Knowledge is power, and the purpose of this book is to tell you what you need to know in order to come to terms with your hypertension, and to live a long and fruitful life.

In the past, the attitude of many doctors toward their patients was patronizing. If you were a patient with hypertension, this might mean that your doctor would be reluctant to tell you what your pressure actually was, and would simply hand you a prescription and tell you to take the pills. Today's patient is no longer a passive recipient of pills, but an educated and informed consumer. The news media all have medical correspondents, and articles describing research findings in medical journals are often featured on the *Seven O'Clock News* and in *USA Today*. This information is often conflicting: on one occasion we are told that vitamin E prevents heart disease and cancer, and on another that it is of no value or possibly even harmful.

The practice of medicine is undergoing major changes. The advent of managed care is producing pressure on doctors to increase their productivity, which means seeing more patients in less time. As a result of this, your questions, such as whether you should take vitamin E, are likely to go unanswered— Next patient, please.

My reason for writing this book was to try to provide answers to questions that my patients commonly ask me about their high blood pressure, but which I am often too busy to answer fully. I can offer no quick fix or magic cure, but I can give you a balanced view of the facts.

There is in fact a lot that you can do to mitigate the effects of high blood pressure and its consequences. Since it doesn't make you feel ill, and won't necessarily have any adverse effects on your general state of health or life expectancy, the first thing to be decided is whether you need do anything at all. One high reading taken in your doctor's office on a day when you're hurried and hassled does not signify that you're going to need to take expensive medication and eat bland food for the rest of your days. One of the themes of this book is that your blood pressure is continually changing, and that to get an accurate assessment of your level of risk, it's usually necessary to take many readings over a prolonged period of time before reaching a decision. Not all of these readings need be taken by a physician, and I advocate the use of self-measurement of blood pressure at home or in the workplace. There are two reasons for this: one is that it provides a convenient and economical way of getting a large number of readings, and the other is that in many people going to the doctor's office for a blood pressure check actually increases the pressure, leading to the phenomenon of "white-coat hypertension."

Another theme of the book is that your blood pressure level needs to be seen in its proper context, which is you, the individual. High blood pressure is important because it may increase your risk of getting heart disease or having a stroke, but it's only one of several risk factors for these conditions. What really matters is not how high your blood pressure is, but how high your chance of getting sick is. The other factors that determine your level of risk depend on who you are and what you do. If you're a premenopausal woman your risk is lower than if you're a man of the same age and with the same blood pressure, and if you're a nonsmoker your risk is lower than if you smoke.

The book is divided into two parts. The first, "Understanding High Blood Pressure," describes what high blood pressure is, how it interacts with other risk factors for cardiovascular disease, what its consequences are, and how they vary in different people. The second, "What You Can Do About High Blood Pressure," describes ways in which you can most effectively deal with it. This may mean taking medication, but there are also lifestyle changes that may enable you to avoid the need for it, or at any rate minimize the amount that you need to take.

A third major theme is that the approach to managing hypertension also needs to be made on an individualized basis. What works well in one case may be useless in another. A good example of this is salt restriction. Conventional wisdom has it that anyone with high blood pressure should be on a low-salt diet, whereas in fact we know that less than half of hypertensive individuals change their blood pressure when they change their salt intake. These people are referred to as being "salt-sensitive"; for the rest, there is no good reason to throw out the salt-shaker. The same is true of medications, where the old adage that one man's meat is another man's poison still holds true.

PART ONE

UNDERSTANDING HIGH BLOOD PRESSURE

CHAPTER ONE

SOME BASIC FACTS ABOUT HIGH BLOOD PRESSURE

Everybody knows that high blood pressure is bad, but most people have only a hazy idea as to why, and what the term really means. In fact, all of us have high blood pressure some of the time, and we wouldn't be able to function if we didn't. High blood pressure is of concern only when it persists for long periods of time, and its adverse effects actually take many years to develop. It's very common: according to official government figures it affects 50 million people in the United States. The other name for it is hypertension, a word that often causes confusion. People who have high blood pressure are not particularly "hyper" or tense, in the usual sense of the word, and the term simply refers to the increased tension, or pressure, in the arteries.

The arteries are the elastic tubes that carry blood from the heart to the tissues. They are configured like a tree; the central trunk, or aorta, leaves the heart, and then branches repeatedly. Very small branches, which are visible only under a microscope, are called arterioles. They have muscle cells in their walls, so that they can constrict and dilate, and hence direct the flow of blood to where it is most needed. The arterioles branch into even finer vessels, called capillaries, which form a delicate mesh that supplies the tissues with oxygen and other nutrients. For the blood to be able to circulate properly, a certain level of pressure is needed to force it through the arterioles and capillaries.

It's important to realize that the blood pressure is continually varying, in order to meet the ever changing needs of our bodies. This was noticed on the very first occasion that blood pressure was measured, by an English priest named Stephen Hales in the year 1733. He inserted a long glass tube into the artery of a horse's neck, and found that the blood reached a height of eight feet in the tube. Not surprisingly, the horse didn't like having its neck punctured in this way, and when it struggled, its blood pressure increased, so the blood in the tube went even higher.

Blood pressure is normally regulated very tightly by the brain. When we're asleep, and our bodies are at rest, we consume less oxygen than when we're awake and active, and so the brain lets the pressure fall to a lower level. At the other extreme, when we're exercising, our muscles need a greater supply of blood to keep them going, and the pressure goes up. The highest pressures of all are seen in weight lifters, in whom the blood pressure may reach three times its normal resting level. There's a good reason for this. When you're holding up a barbell, your arm muscles are contracting for as long as you're holding, and the contraction of the muscles squeezes the arteries and capillaries supplying them, hence tending to shut off their blood supply. The brain overcomes this by signaling the heart to pump in the blood at a higher pressure, thus keeping the arteries open, and enabling the muscles to contract longer. Surges of blood pressure are thus quite normal during either mental or physical activity.

WHAT THE NUMBERS MEAN: SYSTOLIC AND DIASTOLIC PRESSURE

You probably recognize the numbers 120/80 (pronounced "one twenty over eighty") as a normal blood pressure. But why two numbers? The explanation is quite simple. Your heart beats about 70 times a minute, and with each beat blood is pumped into the arteries. As this happens, the pressure inside the arteries goes up, until the end of that heartbeat. The peak level of pressure is called the systolic pressure, because "systole" (pronounced "sist-ol-ly") is the technical term for a heartbeat. Then the heart relaxes, and begins filling with blood for the next beat. This period is called "diastole." While this is happening the pressure in the arteries starts to fall and reaches a minimum level just before the next heartbeat, which is the diastolic pressure. So the number 120 refers to the systolic pressure, and 80 to the diastolic pressure. Each heartbeat produces a slightly different pressure, but usually the two numbers go up and down together.

All measurements have to be expressed in units, which may, for example, be pounds (for weights) or inches (for lengths). The pressure in your car tire is measured in pounds per square inch, but for blood pressure we use millimeters of mercury, usually abbreviated as mm Hg (Hg is the shortened version of the Latin name for mercury). The reasons for using mm Hg are both historical and practical. The pressure gauge used by doctors to measure blood pressure is called a sphygmomanometer, which has a column of mercury, the height of which is recorded in millimeters, and is a measure of the pressure inside the cuff (as explained below).

How Blood Pressure Is Measured

The traditional method of measuring blood pressure is with a sphygmomanometer and a stethoscope. The way it works is as follows: The cloth cuff that is wrapped around your upper arm contains a rubber bag, which can be pumped up with air by squeezing a rubber bulb. The bag is also connected via a tube to the column of mercury, which measures the air pressure in the bag. To take a reading of the blood pressure, the cuff is pumped up to a pressure of about 200 mm Hg. This is nearly always higher than the systolic pressure, so that it completely shuts off the circulation of blood in the arm. Then the valve on the rubber bulb is opened a little, and the air in the bag is allowed to leak out and gradually lower the pressure in the cuff. While this is happening the person taking the pressure listens with a stethoscope placed on the elbow crease, just below the cuff. When the cuff pressure is greater than the systolic pressure, there's no flow of blood and nothing to hear. But as the pressure is reduced, it gets to a point at which the systolic pressure in the artery is higher than the cuff pressure, so the artery starts to open and blood to flow. Each spurt of blood makes a whooshing sound, which can be heard with the stethoscope. As the cuff pressure is reduced further, the sounds get louder and last longer, but as the cuff pressure approaches the diastolic pressure they start to fade away. The point at which they finally disappear is the diastolic pressure. It may seem puzzling why the sounds come and go in this way, but when the flow of blood in the artery is not interrupted by the occlusion produced by the cuff, it's quite smooth and makes no noise. What we hear when the cuff pressure is between systolic and diastolic pressure is partly the sound of the artery opening and closing, as the pressure inside it is either greater or less than the cuff pressure compressing it, and partly the sound of turbulent flow. Incidentally, you can also hear sounds of blood flowing when an artery is partly blocked by plaque, in this case because the narrowing in the artery causes turbulence. Part of the physical exam (described in Chapter 16) is listening over the large arteries in the neck for sounds of obstruction.

HOW BLOOD PRESSURE IS REGULATED

Some appreciation of the complex ways in which blood pressure is normally controlled by the body may be helpful in understanding how the different classes of blood-pressure-lowering medications work. A useful analogy for understanding the basics of blood pressure regulation is a garden hose. The water pressure can be increased in two ways—either by opening the faucet and pumping more water through, or by tightening the nozzle and increasing the resistance to the outflow of water. In exactly the same way, the blood pressure is dependent on two factors, the amount of blood being pumped by the heart (the cardiac output) and the resistance to flow (the peripheral resistance). The latter is regulated largely by the caliber of the small arteries (arterioles), which have muscle fibers in their walls, and like the nozzle on the garden hose can constrict and dilate. This means that when your blood pressure goes up it can do so in three ways: by an increase in the cardiac output, by constriction of the arterioles, or by a combination of the two. When you exercise, your pressure goes up because of an increased cardiac output—the muscles need a greater flow of blood. If you put your hand into iced water your pressure also goes up, but in this case it's purely from constriction of the arterioles.

The brain plays a major role in the regulation of the circulation, through two sets of nerves which act as the yin and yang of circulatory control. One, the sympathetic nervous system, causes the heart to speed up, while the other, the parasympathetic system, makes it slow down. This dual control system allows for very fine tuning of the heart. Both systems are normally switched on: when our heart rate starts to go up at the beginning of exercise it does so by a combination of decreased parasympathetic and increased sympathetic nerve activity. The parasympathetic nerves are mainly involved in the regulation of the heart, while the sympathetic nervous system also controls the tone of the blood vessels, and mediates the "fight-or-flight response," characterized by an increased cardiac output and blood pressure. This is something we all recognize and is experienced as pounding of the heart, sweating, and anxiety. In evolutionary terms this was the appropriate preparation for vigorous physical exercise, whether it be fighting or fleeing from a foe. In modern times our threats are more often psychologi-cal than physical, and this pattern of response may be less appropriate for dealing with them.

The sympathetic nerves transmit their message to the muscle cells of the heart and arteries by releasing a chemical called norepinephrine from the nerve terminals, which rest on the surface of the muscle cells of the heart and arterioles. The norepinephrine molecules latch on to specific receptor sites on the membrane of the muscle cells, which then send a chemical signal to the inside of the cell to initiate the process of contraction. These receptors are called adrenergic receptors (in Europe norepinephrine and epinephrine are called noradrenaline and adrena-line, hence adrenergic), and are of two sorts—alpha and beta. The alpha receptors are mainly situated on the muscle cells in the walls of the arte-rioles, and when stimulated cause the muscle to contract, and hence the arteriole to constrict. Beta receptors are located in several different sites, the most important ones being in the heart, where they stimulate both the strength and speed of contraction, and in the kidney, where they stimulate the release of renin, which is also important in the regu-lation of blood pressure, as described below.

The adrenergic receptors are the targets for two classes of blood-pressure-lowering medications, the alpha and beta blocking agents. Both types work on the same general principle: they have some struc-tural similarity to norepinephrine, which enables them to bind to the adrenergic receptors, but unlike norepinephrine, they do not stimulate the receptor to trigger muscle contraction, and they also prevent the norepinephrine from stimulating the receptors. Hence the term *block-ing agents*. The net effect of both alpha and beta blockers is to lower blood pressure, alpha blockers by dilating the arterioles, and beta block-ers by lowering cardiac output and shutting off renin release.

The muscle cells in the arterioles are structurally and functionally dif-ferent from those in the heart and the muscles in the rest of our body, and are referred to as smooth muscle cells. Their contraction depends on the amount of calcium inside the cell, and in fact the contractile process is triggered by a small amount of calcium passing into the cell through minute pores called calcium channels. The entrance to these channels can be blocked by another group of agents, the calcium-channel blockers, which effectively paralyze the smooth muscle cells.

Another major mechanism for controlling blood pressure is the renin-angiotensin system. Renin is a chemical that is secreted by the kidney, and circulates in the blood. It has no effects on blood pressure itself, but it leads to the formation of another inert chemical—angiotensin I. As it circulates through the lung angiotensin I is converted into angiotensin II by angiotensin converting enzyme. Angiotensin II exerts a very powerful constrictor effect on the arterioles, and thus can raise the blood pressure. It has a second effect, however, which makes it even more potent. It acts on the adrenal gland to release a hormone called aldosterone, which in turn acts on the kidney and causes it to retain sodium. This also tends to raise the blood pressure. One of the normal functions of the renin-angiotensin system is as a defense mechanism to maintain the blood pressure in situations such as hemorrhage or extreme salt depletion. A low blood pressure and a low amount of salt passing through the kidney are two of the three factors that stimulate the kidney to release renin, the third being the sympathetic nervous system.

WHY IS HIGH BLOOD PRESSURE SO BAD?

Everyone has high blood pressure some of the time, and it causes a problem only when it stays high for long periods. Even then, there are many people who live normal lives with high blood pressure, and never know they have it. Unfortunately, not all are so lucky, and the reason doctors are concerned about high blood pressure is that it increases the risk of a number of serious events, chiefly strokes and heart attacks. Even if these do occur, however, it may be only after ten or twenty years of the pressure being high.

The damage caused by high blood pressure is of three general sorts. The first is the one everyone thinks of—bursting a blood vessel. While this is dramatic and disastrous when it happens, it's actually the least common of the three problems. It occurs most frequently in the blood vessels of the brain, where the smaller arteries may develop a weak spot, called an aneurysm. This is an area where the wall is thinner than normal and a bulge develops. When there is a sudden surge of pressure the aneurysm may burst, resulting in bleeding into the tissues of the brain, and hence a stroke.

Aneurysms can also develop in the largest blood vessel in the body, the aorta. Here they gradually enlarge over a period of several years, and because they are so large (sometimes as big as a grapefruit) they can often be detected before they start to leak, and can be treated surgically.

The second adverse consequence of high blood pressure is that it accelerates the deposition of cholesterol plaque (atheroma) in the arteries. This, too, takes many years to develop, but is very difficult to detect until it causes a major blockage. It affects mainly the larger arteries, but its deposition is not uniform. It accumulates most where an artery divides into two smaller branches. The blood flow is normally smooth in the arteries, but where they divide it becomes turbulent, and this turbulence is thought to damage the delicate lining of the arteries. Wherever this occurs, cholesterol deposits are more likely to accumulate. The most important sites to be affected are the heart, where atheroma causes angina and heart attacks; the brain, where it causes strokes; the kidneys, where it causes renal failure (and can also make the blood pressure go even higher); and the legs, where it causes a condition known as intermittent claudication, which means pain during walking. For some unknown reason, it never affects the arteries in the arms. This process is described in more detail in the next chapter.

Third, high blood pressure puts a strain on the heart: because it has to work harder than normal its muscle enlarges, just as does any other muscle that is used excessively. This is not necessarily bad, and athletes such as marathon runners have enlarged hearts (sometimes referred to as athlete's heart). In their case the enlargement occurs primarily because the heart has to be able to pump a bigger volume of blood, as opposed to pumping the blood at a higher pressure, so the chamber of the heart enlarges without the walls getting any thicker. In people with high blood pressure the volume of the heart doesn't change very much, but the thickness of the muscle increases. This can now be measured very accurately by a technique called "echocardiography," which is described in Chapter 16. Thickening of the heart muscle is bad because the muscle outgrows its blood supply, rendering it more susceptible to the effects of atheroma narrowing the coronary arteries, which supply the heart.

IS HIGH BLOOD PRESSURE A DISEASE?

Not really. The word *disease* generally implies sickness and an inability to function properly. The vast majority of people with high blood pressure are not sick in this sense: they have no symptoms, they don't look sick, and they can do the same things as anybody else. It's only when blood pressure gets to very high levels (technically referred to as malignant hypertension) that it makes people feel sick. For those less severely affected, high blood pressure is important merely because it imposes a little extra wear and tear on the circulation. It's more appropriate to regard it as a risk factor, as described below.

DOES HIGH BLOOD PRESSURE AFFECT MY ABILITY TO WORK?

Since high blood pressure causes no symptoms or disability, the logical answer to this question should be no. Unfortunately, many doctors do not follow this logic, and may recommend that people with high blood pressure should not be hired for a job, on the grounds that they are at increased risk of having a heart attack, or perhaps because they think that the stress of the job will raise the blood pressure even more.

In a recent survey of physicians who were members of the American Occupational Medicine Association, all of whom did preemployment medical examinations for corporations, Dr. Michael Murphy found that two thirds of the physicians would exclude people from working for the company because of hypertension. When asked what level of diastolic blood pressure would be needed for the applicant to be rejected, the answers given by the physicians ranged from 90 to 130 mm Hg.

These findings are worrying because they suggest that there is a potential bias in the attitude of many physicians toward hypertensive patients, and the wide range of blood pressures used as the cutoff point for employment indicates that these decisions are based on the whims of the individual doctors, rather than on any scientific basis. I very much doubt if the same physicians would preclude applicants because they smoked or had a high blood cholesterol. A recently enacted law, the Americans with Disabilities Act, should fortunately make this less of a problem in the future, since it prohibits preemployment medical examinations by companies with more than 15 employees.

ARE THERE DIFFERENT TYPES OF HIGH BLOOD PRESSURE?

Yes. High blood pressure can be classified in two ways, one according to how severe it is (mainly a question of how high the blood pressure is), and the other according to what's causing it. About 95 percent of people with high blood pressure have what is known as *essential hypertension*, which is really a fancy way of saying that it just happens, and we don't know why. The other 5 percent of cases have *secondary hypertension*, where there is an identifiable and usually correctable cause. The commonest of these is renovascular hypertension, where there is narrowing of the artery to one or both kidneys. Other less common causes of secondary hypertension are small tumors of the adrenal glands which secrete blood-pressure-raising chemicals (hormones) into the bloodstream.

The term *essential hypertension* is not a very specific one. It is thought that hypertension is the end result of a number of different factors that make the blood pressure go up, and it is probable that different mechanisms are important in different individuals. This may explain why a particular type of treatment may work very well in one person, but not at all in another.

Classification of hypertension by its severity is somewhat arbitrary, because there's no precise level of pressure above which it suddenly becomes dangerous. For no particularly good reason, blood pressure has traditionally been classified according to the height of the diastolic pressure, although the systolic pressure is probably more important in determining the level of risk. Someone whose diastolic pressure runs between 90 and 95 mm Hg may be regarded as having borderline hypertension; when it's between 95 and 110 mm Hg it's moderate; and at any higher levels it's severe. The most dangerous type is called malignant hypertension, which is regarded as an acute emergency requiring immediate treatment in hospital. Whatever the underlying cause, when the blood pressure reaches a certain level for a sufficient length of time it sets off a vicious cycle of damage to the heart, brain, and kidneys, resulting in further elevation of the pressure. Not surprisingly, if untreated, it can rapidly be fatal. Because more people are treated nowadays than before, malignant hypertension is not common, and is mainly seen in people who have not had access to medical care.

White-coat (or office) hypertension is a term used to describe people whose blood pressure is high only in a doctor's office. It is dealt with more fully in Chapter 10.

Systolic hypertension is seen mainly in people over the age of 65, and is characterized by a high systolic but normal diastolic pressure (a reading of 170/80 mm Hg would be typical). It's caused by an age-related loss of elasticity of the major arteries, and is discussed in Chapter 12.

Labile hypertension is a commonly used but inappropriate term for describing high blood pressure that is unusually labile or variable. In fact, just about everyone has labile blood pressure.

RISK FACTORS—THE BIG THREE

Stroke and heart disease are the major causes of death and disability in developed countries, and there are several factors (called risk factors) that make them more likely to occur. Some are things that we can't do anything about, like our age and gender. Older people are more likely to have strokes and heart attacks than younger ones, and men are at greater risk than women. The most important ones that we can do something about are what may be called the Big Three—high blood pressure, high blood cholesterol, and smoking. All of these are quantitative—that is, the more you have of them, the greater your risk. There's no level of blood pressure at which the risk suddenly increases, but it's generally accepted that when the pressure is more than 140/90 mm Hg it begins to be of some concern, and when it's more than 160/100 mm Hg it's definitely too high.

Another important aspect of these risk factors is that they interact with one another. If you're a 50-year-old man and have a systolic blood pressure of 165 mm Hg and a normal cholesterol (185), you have a 5.2 in 100 chance of having a heart attack in the next six years, and if you have a cholesterol of 285 and a normal blood pressure (120) you have a 6.4 in 100 chance. But if you have both a blood pressure of 165 and a cholesterol of 285 your risk is now 10.6 in 100. And if on top of all that you're a smoker, your risk goes up to 15.7 in 100.

HOW DO I KNOW WHEN MY BLOOD PRESSURE IS HIGH?

For the most part you can't tell if you have high blood pressure, and most hypertensive people have no symptoms. So the only way to find out if it's high is to have it measured. This statement may come as a surprise, because many people are convinced that they can tell when their pressure is high. It's certainly true that when you get angry or anxious you may feel yourself tensing up, and your heart pounding. You may even go red in the face, something that's often erroneously associated with high blood pressure. And you're right: your pressure is likely to be high at such times. But that's perfectly normal, and unless you spend your life being permanently angry, which fortunately most of us don't, it doesn't mean much. High blood pressure is of concern only when it's still high when you are not angry or tense.

WHAT ARE THE SYMPTOMS?

Usually, there are no specific symptoms that indicate someone has high blood pressure. But some population surveys have shown that a wide variety of common symptoms, such as sleep disturbance, emotional upsets, and dry mouth, are slightly commoner in people with higher pressures. The differences are small, however. Going red in the face, or feeling flushed, is not indicative of high blood pressure.

HEADACHE AND HIGH BLOOD PRESSURE

If you asked a hundred people what is the commonest symptom of high blood pressure, the chances are that the majority would say headache. In fact, not only do most people with high blood pressure not have headaches any more than the rest of us, but when they do, it's usually not from the blood pressure. Merely having a high level of blood pressure inside your head does not normally produce any symptoms; if you lift a heavy weight, your pressure may go up to 300 mm Hg, but you don't get a headache.

What can cause headache is muscle tension. Any muscle that is tensed for long enough starts to hurt, and chronic tension in the scalp or neck muscles is a very common cause of headache. A study conducted many years ago shed some very interesting light on the relationship between headache and high blood pressure. Out of 104 people who had high blood pressure but were unaware of it, only 3 volunteered that they had headaches, although another 14 admitted it when asked. But of 96 people who had been told that they had high blood pressure, 71 said they had headaches. The simplest explanation for this finding is that being told that you have high blood pressure makes you start to worry, and that this in turn causes the headaches.

There is a much smaller number of patients, mostly with very high pressures, in whom headaches are directly related to the height of the blood pressure. In such individuals treating the blood pressure will relieve the symptoms.

WHICH IS MORE IMPORTANT—SYSTOLIC OR DIASTOLIC PRESSURE?

It is a common misconception that diastolic pressure (the lower of the two numbers) is more important as a predictor of risk than systolic pressure (the higher number) is. The reason for this is partly historical. The first large-scale trial of the effectiveness of blood-pressure-lowering medication in preventing strokes and heart attacks, the Veterans Administration trial conducted by Dr. Edward Fries, selected patients for the trial solely on the basis of their diastolic pressures. Since that time, other similar trials have followed the same practice, so most of our knowledge about the benefits of treating high blood pressure is based on the level of diastolic pressure. But epidemiological studies of the risks associated with a particular level of blood pressure have shown that of the two measures, systolic pressure is slightly more important. This is of special significance in older people, who often have a normal diastolic but raised systolic pressure. Such people are at increased risk, and a recent study has shown that this risk can be reduced by treatment, as described in Chapter 12.

DEFINING HIGH BLOOD PRESSURE

It may come as a surprise to learn that experts are still unable to agree on an exact definition of high blood pressure. The problem is that any definition is quite arbitrary, because there's no clear separation between what is a "normal" as opposed to a "high" pressure. In general, the higher the pressure, the worse are the consequences. It's the same problem as trying to define when someone is fat as opposed to thin, or tall as opposed to short. Understanding this point is very important, because high blood pressure is not a condition that you either have or don't have (in contrast to cancer, for example). In other words, it's a quantitative rather than a qualitative disorder.

All the experts agree that a blood pressure below 140/90 mm Hg is normal, and that a pressure above 160/100 mm Hg is too high. The "gray zone," where there is genuine disagreement among doctors, is a pressure that falls somewhere in between these two levels. Ideally, if your pressure is in this borderline range, your doctor's decision on whether you need treatment should take into consideration whether you have other risk factors. This issue is discussed in more detail in Chapter 22.

CAN HIGH BLOOD PRESSURE BE TREATED?

The good news is that high blood pressure is eminently treatable. The objective of treatment is not simply to lower the blood pressure, but to prevent its consequences, such as strokes and heart attacks. The benefits of treatment were first convincingly demonstrated in a landmark Veterans Administration study conducted by Dr. Edward Fries, the first results of which were published in 1967. This study included 143 men with severe hypertension, who had diastolic pressures between 115 and 129 mm Hg. Half of the 143 men were treated with medication to lower the blood pressure, while the others received inert placebo pills. After only one and a half years, the results were quite clear: in the untreated group, 4 men had died, and 23 had developed "complications" (a medical euphemism for strokes, heart attacks, and other catastrophic consequences of high blood pressure), while in the treated group none had died, and only 2 had developed complications. A second report, published in 1970, found that in 380 men with less severe hypertension (diastolic pressures between 90 and 114 mm Hg), three and a half years of treatment cut the rate of complications by half, and there were 19 deaths in the untreated group, but only 14 in the treated group. Since that time several studies have shown that treating patients with milder forms of hypertension (diastolic pressures between 90 and 105 mm Hg) is also beneficial, although the results are much less dramatic.

SUMMARY

• Blood pressure goes up and down with each heartbeat, and is expressed as two numbers, the systolic and diastolic pressures, which are the upper and lower number, respectively. The normal range is from 100 to 140 for systolic, and 70 to 90 for diastolic pressure. A typical reading would be 120 (systolic) and 80 (diastolic), which would be described as "120 over 80," and written as 120/80.

• Our blood pressure is continually changing; when we exercise it can go as high as 200/100, and when we sleep as low as 90/50.

• High blood pressure is defined as a persistently high level (measured on several occasions), typically more than 140/90.

• High blood pressure usually causes no symptoms, but increases the risk of getting cardiovascular disease such as heart attacks and strokes. Lowering the pressure can reduce these risks.

• The other two major risk factors for cardiovascular disease are cigarette smoking and a high blood cholesterol.

• In general, the higher the pressure the greater the risk. Both systolic and diastolic pressures are important, but systolic is more so.

CHAPTER TWO

DISEASE OF THE ARTERIES— CHOLESTEROL AND ATHEROSCLEROSIS

Although high blood pressure and arterial disease, or atherosclerosis, are separate processes, they occur together with such frequency that they may be considered to be two sides of the same coin. High blood pressure accelerates the development of atherosclerosis, but it is only one of many causes. In this chapter I will focus on one of the other major risk factors for atherosclerosis—high blood cholesterol and related disorders. This is a complex and controversial story, which is played out in the pages of the national press. Here are two examples: For years we have been told that we should be striving to keep our cholesterol levels as low as possible, but recently there has been the heretical suggestion that very low cholesterol levels may also be bad. And margarine was always thought to be a good substitute for butter, but now this too is in doubt.

What Is Atherosclerosis?

Athero is the Greek word for gruel, and *sclerosis* means hardening; that describes the process pretty well. It's often referred to as hardening of the arteries, but it would be more appropriate to think of it as a series of deposits that gradually develop on the insides of the vessels, and can eventually block them off completely. In Western societies atherosclerosis is very common: in the Framingham Heart Study about 70 percent of men and women over the age of 65 have deposits in their carotid arteries that can be detected by a simple noninvasive test. (Framingham is a suburb of Boston, and much of our knowledge of the epidemiology of cardiovascular disease comes from this study of its inhabitants, which has been going on for about forty years.)

Atherosclerosis starts in childhood, and gradually develops over fifty years or so before causing any problems. It's first detectable as streaks of fat in the abdominal aorta (the large artery that supplies the blood flow to our legs), and then gradually spreads to involve the arteries going to our kidneys, neck, brain, and heart. It is deposited as plaques, which are like lumps of candle wax embedded in the walls of the arteries. The plaques form in certain favored spots, particularly where a large artery divides into two branches. Nothing happens until the plaque has narrowed the inside of the artery by at least 50 percent. When it gets to be more than that it starts to interfere with the blood flow through the artery, which is when the troubles start. If the obstruction first develops in one of the arteries supplying the heart (the coronary arteries), it is manifested as angina. The blood supply to the heart may be adequate at rest, but inadequate during exercise, when the heart muscle is working harder and using more oxygen. More disastrously, a blood clot may form on the plaque, completely plugging the artery and leading to a heart attack.

The process begins with the seepage of cholesterol from the blood into the inner layers of the arterial wall, with the formation of what are called fatty streaks. Another factor is injury to the endothelium, which is a thin layer of cells lining the inner wall of the artery. This injury may be of chemical origin (for example, nicotine), or it may be mechanical (the wear and tear of blood flow, particularly at branch points in the vessels where the flow becomes turbulent). When, as a result of these injuries, the endothelium gets torn, platelets and white cells from the blood stick to the bare area. Platelets are the smallest of the circulating blood cells, whose main function is to control damage by sticking to any injured area of the arterial wall and initiating the clotting process. If the injuries continue, some of these cells may burrow into the wall of the artery and start to form a local swelling, which begins to encroach on the lumen of the artery, that is, the space through which the blood flows. More cholesterol accumulates in these plaques, and can be seen as crystals when examined under the microscope. The protruding plaque causes further turbulence of the blood flowing past it, and the stretching of the endothelium covering the plaque makes it liable to further damage.

It used to be thought that this process goes on gradually over many years, like the furring of a water pipe, but we now know that it's much more episodic, going in fits and starts. Eventually a plaque may rupture, setting off a blood clot on the wounded area. If this is big enough to oc-clude the artery completely, a stroke or heart attack may be the result.

THE LIPID HYPOTHESIS—LINKING DIETARY FAT TO ATHEROSCLEROSIS AND CARDIOVASCULAR DISEASE

The idea that a fatty diet might be related to atherosclerosis began in an unlikely place—on the island of Java. In 1916, a Dutch medical practi-tioner named Dr. de Langen suggested that the Javanese people had very little atherosclerosis because they ate little food containing fat and cholesterol. And when they began to eat a European-style diet that was rich in animal fat their cholesterol levels went up. Since that time his ob-servation has been abundantly confirmed, and surveys from 30 countries all over the world have shown that the death rate from coronary heart disease is closely linked to the dietary intake of cholesterol and saturated fat. The countries at the top of the list are Finland, New Zealand, the United Kingdom, and the United States—all meat- and cheese-eating countries. The countries where the heart attack rates are much lower are Portugal and the Mediterranean ones such as Spain and Greece, where the diet is rich in olive oil, and Japan, where people eat a lot of fish.

There are some notable exceptions to this, such as France, where coronary disease is surprisingly rare; this is discussed in Chapter 4. An-other population that doesn't fit this pattern is the Eskimos from Green-land, who eat a very-high-fat diet, but don't get heart disease. This is because they also eat a lot of fish, which has a protective effect, also de-scribed in Chapter 4. During World War II, when Norway was occupied by the Germans, the death rate from heart disease decreased dramati-cally. The food shortages meant that very little meat was available, so people ate fish instead.

Nowadays, just about everybody agrees that eating a diet high in satu-rated fat raises your blood cholesterol level, and that this leads to the de-velopment of coronary heart disease. This sequence is often referred to as the lipid hypothesis, which is accepted as gospel by organizations such as the American Heart Association, and forms the basis of their recommendations for a "heart-healthy" diet. (*Lipid* is a term that is used to describe fat and cholesterol.)

THE LIPID HYPOTHESIS

High intake of saturated fat → *Raised blood cholesterol* → *Coronary heart disease*

However, it's also important to realize that a high blood cholesterol level doesn't happen only because you eat a lot of fat and cholesterol. Your body also makes cholesterol, and there are some people who inherit a tendency to make excessive amounts, and who may have heart attacks while still children.

As a general rule of thumb, for every 1 percent rise in blood cholesterol, there is a 2 to 3 percent rise in the chances of getting coronary heart disease.

WHAT IS CHOLESTEROL, AND WHERE DOES IT COME FROM?

Cholesterol gets such a bad press that you might think it is a poison, but in actual fact it is an essential component of cell walls. About three quarters of the cholesterol in our bodies is manufactured in the liver. It's not soluble in blood, so it has to be transported by combining with special transporter proteins, called lipoproteins. There are three principal kinds of these: high-density, low-density, and very-low-density lipoproteins, which are usually referred to as HDL, LDL, and VLDL. Most of the cholesterol in the blood is carried by HDL and LDL. When you have your blood cholesterol checked, it can be measured either as the total amount or as the amounts of LDL and HDL. Some of the circulating cholesterol is taken up by the tissues to be used as building blocks for making cell membranes and hormones (chemical messengers). Much of it is recycled to the liver, where it shuts off further production of cholesterol. This requires the cholesterol molecules to attach themselves to specific receptors on the surface of the liver cells before they can pass through the cell wall. In 1985 two American researchers, Drs. Michael Brown and Joseph Goldstein, were awarded the Nobel Prize in medicine for discovering that the reason some children are born with a hereditary form of very high cholesterol levels, resulting in heart attacks before they reach adulthood, is that they lack these receptors on their liver cells. This means that no cholesterol is recycled into the liver cells, which consequently increase their production of cholesterol. Furthermore, the liver is the only organ that can excrete cholesterol (as bile), so this disposal route is also blocked. The end result is that the blood cholesterol reaches very high levels, and the excess is deposited as plaque in the arteries.

In its native state, cholesterol is relatively harmless, and is an essential component of cell membranes and body chemicals. However, if it comes into contact with free radicals (described in Chapter 24) it becomes *oxidized* cholesterol (oxidized means combined with oxygen), in which form it is taken up by cells of the arterial walls and deposited as plaque. The importance of oxidation was first demonstrated by Dr. Daniel Steinberg at the University of Southern California at San Diego. One of his experiments was conducted in a special strain of rabbits that are genetically predisposed to developing atheroma in the form of fatty streaks lining their arteries. One group of rabbits was fed a powerful antioxidant drug called probucol, which also has a weak cholesterol-lowering effect. Another was given a second drug, lovastatin, which lowered the cholesterol to the same extent, but which is not an antioxidant. The rabbits that were given probucol developed only half the number of fatty streaks, which could be attributed to its preventing the oxidation of cholesterol.

LDL CHOLESTEROL ("BAD CHOLESTEROL")

Our cholesterol comes from two sources—what we eat and what we make—and it is transported in the blood by hooking on to a protein called low-density lipoprotein (LDL). Measuring LDL cholesterol gives the most accurate estimate of how much cholesterol you have. The higher your LDL cholesterol, the higher your risk of vascular disease, so it's often referred to as the "bad cholesterol." The factors that affect your LDL level are listed in Table 2.1 (note that different medications can either raise or lower LDL).

Table 2.1. Factors Affecting LDL

RAISE LDL	LOWER LDL
Saturated fat	Polyunsaturated fat
Medications	Monounsaturated fat
	Dietary fiber
	Medications

What Should My Cholesterol Be? The National Cholesterol Education Program recently issued a set of guidelines for cholesterol levels. In the United States, the levels are usually expressed as mg/dl, which means the number of milligrams of cholesterol in one deciliter of blood. (A different method is used in Europe.) A few years ago most doctors thought that levels of 250 mg/dl were fine, but over the past few years the acceptable levels have grown progressively lower. The latest ones are shown in Table 2.2.

Table 2.2. Classification of Cholesterol Levels

CLASSIFICATION	TOTAL CHOLESTEROL	LDL CHOLESTEROL
Desirable	Below 199	Below 129
Borderline	200–239	130–159
High	Above 240	Below 160

The National Cholesterol Education Program has also issued a set of guidelines for levels of LDL cholesterol that should be treated, according to whether or not you already have known coronary heart disease. These are shown in Table 2.3.

Table 2.3. NCEP Recommendations for Levels of LDL Cholesterol That Require Treatment

	LEVEL FOR DIET TREATMENT	LEVEL FOR DRUG TREATMENT
No CHD*	Above 160	Above 190
With CHD	Above 130	Above 160

*CHD = coronary heart disease.

HDL CHOLESTEROL ("GOOD CHOLESTEROL")

Although it has been recognized for many years that high HDL is associated with lower risk of heart disease, the official report of the National Cholesterol Education Program published in 1988 made no specific recommendations about the measurement of HDL. One of the chief proponents of its importance has been Dr. William Castelli, who heads the Framingham Heart Study. In people lucky enough to have a very high HDL (85 or more) the risk of heart disease remains less than half the average level even when the LDL is quite high (220). And conversely, when the HDL is very low, the risk may be high even when the LDL is low. In other words, the best predictor of risk is provided by the ratio of the LDL to HDL.

There is a two-way traffic of cholesterol in and out of the tissues; high LDL cholesterol levels in the blood promote the entry of cholesterol into the vessel walls and the formation of atheromatous plaque, while high HDL levels lead to its removal. HDL probably has two other beneficial effects: first, it may inhibit the transformation of LDL cholesterol into its more toxic oxidized form, and second, it may make blood platelets less sticky. All of these actions would tend to retard the formation of atherosclerotic plaque.

Like all the other blood lipids, your HDL is partly determined by your genes, but there are other influences, as shown in Table 2.4.

Table 2.4. Factors Affecting HDL

RAISE HDL	LOWER HDL
Exercise	Physical inactivity
Alcohol	Smoking
Weight loss	Obesity
Medications	Medications
	Low-fat diet

HDL levels are often low in people with a sedentary lifestyle, and high in marathoners. To improve your HDL with exercise, you need to do enough to make you start to lose weight. Another potent way to raise it is to drink alcohol, although few doctors would recommend this as a remedy, because of its other potentially harmful effects. Diet has relatively little effect on HDL, although weight loss, whether produced by diet or exercise, does tend to raise it. Quitting smoking may also help. Some blood-pressure-lowering medications (for example, beta blockers) may lower HDL, but the effect is usually very small, and often transient. There are others that raise it, and these are reviewed in Chapter 22.

The evidence that raising HDL reduces your risk of coronary heart disease comes mainly from two studies. The first was the Coronary Drug Project, which established that nicotinic acid, which raises HDL in addition to lowering triglycerides, can cut the risk of having a heart attack (this is described in more detail in Chapter 24). The second was the Helsinki Trial, which used another HDL-raising medication (gemfibrozil), and reported a reduction in heart attacks of 38 percent. In this study the greatest benefit was seen in patients who started out with a high blood triglyceride and low HDL.

What Should My HDL Cholesterol Be? The higher your HDL level, the lower your risk of coronary heart disease. Typical levels for men are around 45 mg/dl and for women 55 mg/dl. The critical level is generally accepted to be 35 mg/dl, so if you're below this your doctor may recommend treatment.

WHAT IS THE CHOLESTEROL/HDL RATIO?

A very convenient way of expressing your risk of heart disease which takes into account both the total (most of which is the bad, or LDL, cholesterol) and HDL (good) cholesterol is the ratio between the two. If you're a man with a ratio under 4.5, you don't need to worry, although a "perfect" score would be under 3.5. So if your total cholesterol is 200 and your HDL is 50, your ratio is 4, and you're OK. But if your total is 200 and your HDL is 35, your ratio is 5.7, and you may have a problem. As shown in Table 2.5, the ratios are generally lower for women than for men.

The ratio is sometimes expressed as the LDL/HDL ratio, in which case the cutoff point would be 4 for a man and 3 for a woman. It's actually no better than the cholesterol/HDL ratio in terms of predicting who's at risk, and it's more expensive to perform.

Table 2.5. Risk of Heart Disease According to Lipid Ratios

	MEN		WOMEN	
RISK GROUP	Chol/HDL	LDL/HDL	Chol/HDL	LDL/HDL
Below average	3.8 & below	2.3 & below	2.9 & below	2.3 & below
Average	3.9–4.7	2.3–4.9	3.0–3.6	2.3–4.1
Moderate	4.8–5.9	4.9–7.1	3.7–4.6	4.1–5.6
High	6.0 & above	7.2 & above	4.7 & above	5.7 & above

TRIGLYCERIDES

When you eat a fatty meal, much of the fat is absorbed directly into the bloodstream as triglycerides (which is simply the technical name for fat;

see Chapter 4), and it may come as no surprise to learn that having a high triglyceride level in the blood is a risk factor for coronary heart disease. Nevertheless, of the three major lipid components (the other two being LDL and HDL cholesterol) the triglycerides are the least important. The problem in evaluating the role of triglycerides has been that there is a strong association between triglycerides and HDL, such that high triglycerides tend to occur in conjunction with a low HDL, so that it's not clear whether the increased risk is due to the low HDL rather than the high triglycerides. Nevertheless, in the Framingham Heart Study a high triglyceride level in women over the age of 50 does appear to be an independent risk factor.

Triglycerides may be high for a number of reasons, the most important of which are:

- Genetic predisposition
- High fat intake
- Obesity
- Diabetes
- Alcohol

There are a number of genetic conditions that lead to increased triglycerides; they may also be associated with high cholesterol, low HDL, and high blood pressure. The combination of obesity, high triglycerides, and insulin resistance is discussed in Chapter 5. In some people, even moderate alcohol intake can raise triglycerides. One of the side effects of some blood-pressure-lowering medications is to raise triglycerides, which is most noticeable with the diuretics, although the changes are usually quite small.

Because the blood triglyceride level is affected by food, it's important to have your blood tested after you've fasted for at least 12 hours (total cholesterol and HDL cholesterol are less affected).

The treatment of high triglycerides is primarily by diet, and is generally no different from the treatment of high cholesterol—restriction of calorie and fat intake, except that if alcohol is thought to be contributory, it should be restricted as well.

What Should My Triglycerides Be? The first point to make is that routine measurement of triglycerides is not necessary, except that it is needed for the calculation of LDL cholesterol. The upper limit of normal is taken as 200 mg/dl.

How Lipid Levels Are Measured

The conventional method of measuring the levels of cholesterol and other lipids is by taking a venous blood sample. Most laboratories measure total cholesterol, HDL cholesterol, and triglycerides as part of their routine screening test. Since both cholesterol and triglycerides are carried in the blood by being wrapped up in proteins, it is the proteins that are actually measured. The total cholesterol (TC) consists of three major components—LDL, HDL, and VLDL (the lipoprotein-carrying triglyceride). Although LDL is the most important of the three for causing vascular disease, there is no convenient way of measuring it directly, so it has to be estimated from measurements of the others. The formula that is used is

LDL cholesterol = Total cholesterol – HDL cholesterol – Triglycerides ÷ 5

There are also automatic analyses that will give an instantaneous reading of total cholesterol from a small sample of blood taken from a finger stick. They are less accurate than the conventional method, however, and I do not recommend them.

Measuring Your Own Cholesterol

An interesting new development is a kit with which you can measure your cholesterol at home. It's called the Advanced Care Cholesterol Test, and is marketed by Johnson and Johnson. It sells for about $15 in drugstores, and lets you make a single measurement of your total cholesterol. You simply prick your finger, put a drop of blood in a cavity on the device, and read off the value ten minutes later. The test has been shown to be reasonably accurate (to within about 5 percent, or 10 points, of the conventional method).

Do I Need to Fast Before Having a Cholesterol Test?

The lipid component that is most affected by when you last ate is the triglycerides, whose blood levels go up and down according to how much fat is being absorbed from the gut. It is therefore very important to have fasted for at least 12 hours to get a meaningful estimate of your triglyceride level. Since estimating LDL cholesterol also involves knowing the triglyceride value, the same applies to measuring LDL. Total cholesterol and HDL cholesterol are less affected by meals, however.

OUR CHOLESTEROL LEVELS ARE DECLINING

There is no doubt that, as a nation, we have become more health conscious over the years, and one place where this is showing is in our blood cholesterol. For the past thirty years the government has been conducting national health surveys, which have included cholesterol measurements. Table 2.6 shows the results, broken down by race and sex.

Table 2.6. Blood Total Cholesterol Levels in the U.S. Population

	1961	1972	1978	1990
Black men	210	212	208	200
Black women	216	217	213	205
White men	218	213	211	205
White women	223	215	214	205

Source: *Journal of the American Medical Association,* 269: 3015, June 1993.

When these surveys were started they did not include the breakdown of cholesterol into HDL and LDL, which has been done only since 1976. Since that time, however, LDL has declined, while HDL has shown no change. Although the statistics are less clear on this point, the explanation for the change is thought to be a decreased intake of fat in our diets.

Although these changes don't look very dramatic, they may account for part of the decline in deaths from heart disease that has been observed over the same period. Other studies have shown that for each 1 percent decline in cholesterol there is a 2 percent decline in coronary deaths.

IS A VERY LOW CHOLESTEROL DANGEROUS?

Over the past few years, a disturbing but persistent trend has emerged from the results of several large-scale studies that have investigated the effects of lowering cholesterol with medications: even though the number of deaths from heart attacks was reduced, the total mortality was not. This was because there was a larger than expected number of deaths from a variety of causes in the treatment groups, the most prominent of which were suicides and accidents. The same phenomenon was seen in trials in which cholesterol was lowered by diet, so it couldn't be written off as being a side effect of the drugs. But because these numbers were relatively small, and no single cause of death stood out, the experts at first dismissed them as simply being coincidence. Since then a flurry of publications has appeared that has proved beyond reasonable doubt that the experts were wrong. Let's look at some of them.

A group of Swedish investigators examined a set of data that was collected in the county of Värmland in 1964, when cholesterol measurements were made in 27,000 men and the same number of women. The causes of death over the next 20 years were analyzed, and the results showed that people with the lowest cholesterol levels were nearly three times as likely to commit suicide or die from injuries as those with higher levels. A study in California found the same thing, and it has been suggested that having a very low cholesterol may cause a disturbance of brain chemistry that leads to depression. This remains unproven, however.

In 1990 the National Institutes of Health decided to examine the question, and organized a conference of experts from all over the world, who pooled their data to address the issue. The results of 19 studies involving more than 600,000 subjects were examined, from countries including the United States, Japan, Yugoslavia, Israel, and Scotland. They were all epidemiological studies, with measurements made of cholesterol at the start of the study and then ascertainment of the cause of death many years later. Overall, there were 68,406 deaths, of which just under half were from cardiovascular disease. The first analysis looked at overall mortality. In men the highest mortality was seen in those with the highest cholesterol levels (240 or greater)—no surprise here. But it also showed that men with the lowest cholesterol (160 or less) had a higher death rate than men with values between 160 and 200. In other words, the curve relating cholesterol level and death was U-shaped. For cardiovascular deaths there was no U: the lower the cholesterol, the lower the death rate. In women the results were more surprising. The overall death rate was approximately the same, whatever the cholesterol. There was no consistent trend for more cardiovascular deaths at higher levels of cholesterol. Men with low cholesterol had an increased risk of dying from cancer and other causes; in women there was no relationship with cancer deaths, but they also showed a higher death rate from other causes.

These results, which were published in the American Heart Association's prestigious journal *Circulation,* should have been very disturbing for the cholesterol evangelists, who have been advocating that everyone should be trying to keep their cholesterol as low as possible. In fact, the authors of this analysis dodged the issue, and concluded that "definitive interpretation of the associations observed was not possible, although most participants considered it likely that many of the statistical associations of low or lowered cholesterol are explainable by confounding in one form or another." What they meant by this is that you can't tell from this type of analysis which is the chicken and which the egg: Does having a low cholesterol increase your risk of getting cancer, or does cancer lower your cholesterol? There is some evidence for the latter, because people who die from colon cancer tend to show a falling blood cholesterol level in the preceding 10 years.

In other words, you believe statistics only when you want to. In an editorial entitled "Health Policy on Cholesterol: Time to Change Directions" accompanying this article, Dr. Stephen Hulley faced the issue much more directly, and concluded that "we should draw back from universal screening and treatment of blood cholesterol for primary prevention."

My own interpretation of these results is, first, that there's no point in striving to get your total cholesterol below 200, unless you already have heart disease, and second, that women don't need to be so concerned about their cholesterol as men. They should, however, pay attention to their HDL level.

The issue of how much cholesterol should be lowered in people with high levels is discussed further in Chapter 23.

CAN A LOW-FAT DIET PREVENT CORONARY HEART DISEASE?

Epidemiological studies of the relationship between diet and heart disease conducted in many different countries throughout the world have shown that the countries with the lowest rates can be lumped into two groups: those that eat a "Mediterranean diet," such as Greece, Spain, and Italy, and those that eat an "Oriental diet," such as China and Japan.

The factors common to both types of diet are, first, they are low in saturated fat and animal products; second, they are low in processed foods; and third, they are high in grains and vegetables. The big difference between them is in the total fat content: the Mediterranean diet is not low fat, because of the olive oil used in cooking, whereas the Oriental diet is very low in all kinds of fat. The important point about olive oil is that the fat is monounsaturated. The overwhelming evidence is that both of these diets are superior to the typical American or northern European diet.

What is much less firmly established is the benefit to be gained by simply restricting fat intake in the American diet. There is absolutely no dispute that switching to a low-fat diet can lower blood cholesterol levels, although in some people the changes are quite small (see Chapter 18); what is still hotly debated is whether moderate fat restriction can also prevent coronary heart disease. There have been at least 15 randomly controlled studies of the effects of a low-fat diet on heart attacks, ranging in size from 80 to 60,000 men, and with a net fall in blood cholesterol levels ranging from zero to 15 percent. Only 5 of them showed a significant reduction in the rate of heart attacks as a result of changing the diet, and only 3 studies showed a reduction in the overall death rate. Of these 3, 2 included only "high-risk" men, who had already had a heart attack, and all 3 used other interventions (such as quitting smoking) in addition to the dietary change.

Studies using cholesterol-lowering drugs, which can produce bigger falls in blood cholesterol than dietary change, have been more encouraging (see Chapter 23), but until recently there was doubt as to whether taking the drugs will make you live longer. This doubt has now been dispelled, however, since the results of a large Scandinavian study have been published. This showed that a cholesterol-lowering drug given to people who already have heart disease and a high blood cholesterol not only reduces the risk of further heart attacks but also prolongs life.

The bottom line would appear to be this: If you are at very high risk of developing heart disease, or you are already known to have it, your life expectancy and chances of avoiding further trouble will be improved by eating a low-fat diet and making other lifestyle changes. But if you simply have high blood pressure and a high cholesterol, there is no convincing evidence that eating a low-fat diet will make a significant difference. This does not mean that you should take a nihilistic attitude about your diet (see Chapters 18 and 19), but simply avoiding fat is not the answer.

CAN ATHEROSCLEROTIC OBSTRUCTIONS BE DISSOLVED?

Until quite recently it was thought that there was no way, other than by surgery, that atherosclerotic obstructions could be made to go away, and that they would relentlessly continue to enlarge until they throttled the blood flow through the arteries. Happily, it is now clear that this gloomy view was wrong. More than half of a plaque is composed of cholesterol and fats, and it has been shown that these molecules can move backward and forward between the plaque and the blood. This led researchers to speculate that if the blood cholesterol was aggressively lowered, cholesterol might be sucked out of the plaques and shrink them.

There are now at least nine published studies in which this possibility has been systematically examined, and confirmed. The design of these studies has been similar, and has involved a group of patients with proven coronary artery disease, who are randomly allocated to a control group and receive no special cholesterol-lowering treatment, and one or more treatment groups, whose cholesterol is lowered by diet, or drugs, or both. The extent of atherosclerosis is measured by performing angiograms (X rays) of the coronary arteries at the beginning of the study, and a second time after two or three years of treatment. A good example of such a study is the St. Thomas's Atheroma Regression Study (STARS), in which treatment was either a lipid-lowering diet, or diet plus a drug (cholestyramine). The results were encouraging. In the control group (who got no treatment) progression of coronary artery narrowing was observed in 46 percent of cases, while it occurred in only 12 and 15 percent of the treated patients. And improvement in the diameter of the arteries was observed in only 4 percent of the controls, but in 38 and 33 percent of the treated groups. The best results were observed in the group that was treated with both diet and the drug.

The other studies have found generally similar results. In the treated groups the narrowings became on average 2 percent less, whereas in the controls they became 1 percent worse. (Arterial narrowings are normally graded on a percentage score, where 0 percent means no narrowing, and 100 percent means complete blockage of the artery.) These treatment effects sound trivial, but what is really exciting (and also unexpected) is that the number of heart attacks and bypass operations appears to be cut in half as the result of treatment. The numbers are small at present, but are consistent across the different studies.

The explanation that has been proposed to account for the difference between the apparently small effect on the size of the narrowings and the apparently large effect on the occurrence of heart attacks is that the treatment somehow stabilizes the plaques. It is now clear that most major heart attacks are caused when the fibrous cap of a relatively small plaque tears, exposing the tissue underneath. The lining of an artery is normally like the Teflon coating on a nonstick pan: when the Teflon coating is scratched, the food sticks to the pan. When the lining of the artery is torn, a blood clot may form, which can completely plug the artery. Recent research has shown that the plaques that are most likely to tear are the ones where the fibrous cap is sitting on a wobbly blob of cholesterol. Aggressive treatment with lipid-lowering agents sucks out the cholesterol, making the plaque less likely to rupture.

SUMMARY

• The process that leads to disease of the arteries, and that is accelerated by high blood pressure, is called atherosclerosis. It involves the accumulation of cholesterol-rich cells in the wall of the artery. Over many years this can form a plaque that restricts the flow of blood through the artery, and if a blood clot forms on the surface of the plaque, it can block off the artery altogether. This may result in a stroke or heart attack.

• A high blood cholesterol level can accelerate this process; your cholesterol level is influenced partly by what you eat (mainly how much fat and cholesterol), but also by how much cholesterol your body makes, which is determined by your genes.

• There are two sorts of cholesterol, the "bad cholesterol," or LDL (low-density lipoprotein), and the "good cholesterol," or HDL (high-density lipoprotein). A normal total cholesterol is officially defined as 200 or below, with an LDL of 130 or below, and an HDL of 50 or higher.

• Unless you already have heart disease, there is no need to try to lower your total cholesterol below 200, because there is evidence that people with very low cholesterol levels have an increased death rate from noncardiovascular causes. If you do have heart disease, you should try to get it as low as possible.

• Triglycerides (the word means fats) are also commonly measured in blood tests. They are less important as a risk factor for cardiovascular disease than cholesterol is, but ideally should be below 200.

• The progression of atherosclerotic obstructions can be delayed, and to some extent reversed, by eating a low-fat diet and taking cholesterol-lowering medications.

CHAPTER THREE

THE GREAT SALT DEBATE

Of all the potential causes of hypertension, none is more controversial than salt. Restriction of salt intake was the first effective treatment of hypertension, and experts are still sharply divided as to its role. Most doctors now believe that moderate salt restriction helps the majority of patients, while a few believe that it is not only generally ineffective, but also potentially harmful. In this chapter I will try to give you a balanced view of the evidence on both sides.

WHAT IS SALT?

Salt is a substance that is a fundamental component of all animal life and is a chemical combination of two elements, sodium and chlorine, known technically as sodium chloride. All forms of animal life originated in the sea, and it's no coincidence that our bodies have the same concentration of sodium chloride as seawater does. Not all the sodium in our bodies comes from salt, and neither does all the chloride, but salt is the major source of both. It used to be thought that it is only the sodium that is important for blood pressure regulation, but recent studies have shown that the chloride also contributes. If sodium is given without chloride (for example, as sodium phosphate) to salt-depleted hypertensive patients, their blood pressure doesn't go up as much as when they are given sodium chloride.

WHAT IS THE EVIDENCE INCRIMINATING SALT?

The extent to which salt is responsible for high blood pressure is still a matter of controversy, although there are few if any doctors who would say that it is of no importance. The evidence implicating salt is of two main types. First are population studies showing that people who eat more salt are more likely to have high blood pressure than those who eat little, and second are experimental studies of the effects on blood pressure of changing salt intake. The largest of the population studies was called Intersalt and was a survey of 10,000 men and women in 32 countries, which included such diverse populations as Indians living in the jungles of Brazil, natives of Papua New Guinea and Kenya, and people from the United States, China, Russia, and Europe. This study showed that there was, indeed, a relationship between salt intake and blood pressure, but that it was not very strong. Overall, there was a tendency for populations with a higher salt intake to have slightly higher blood pressures, but this was partly because there were four primitive societies which had very low blood pressures and ate practically no salt. Critics said that including these populations was equivalent to loading the dice, since their general lifestyles bore such little resemblance to our own. When their results were left out, the relationship between salt and blood pressure was not nearly so strong, although it was still there. The study would predict that cutting the average American's salt intake in half would lower systolic pressure by about 2 mm Hg and diastolic by 1, a negligible amount.

When salt intake is related to blood pressure in a single population, as has been done in the Framingham Heart Study in the United States, the people with higher blood pressure do not in general consume more salt than those with lower pressure.

Experiments in which people have been fed diets with different amounts of salt have yielded more meaningful information. In people with normal blood pressure very large changes in salt intake usually have very little effect on blood pressure. This is well illustrated by a study conducted in Indianapolis by Dr. Ray Murray on eight healthy volunteers, whose dietary sodium intake was varied from 10 milliequivalents (mEq) per day (virtually salt-free) to 800 mEq (about four times the average intake). To achieve the highest level of salt intake they had to drink salty bouillon between meals and at bedtime. Finally, for the last three days of the study they also had saline solution infused intravenously. Up to a level of salt intake which would normally be regarded as high (nearly 20 grams per day), blood pressure changed by only 2 mm Hg. It was only when really excessive levels were reached that it started to go up, by about 7 mm Hg. In a recent analysis of the results of 33 studies of the effects of salt restriction in patients with mild hypertension, it was concluded that reducing salt intake to 3 grams per day (about a quarter of the normal amount) would lower systolic pressure by about 5 mm Hg on average and diastolic pressure by about 2. These changes are likely to be greater in people with higher pressures. There is general agreement that restricting salt in people with normal blood pressure has no consistent effect.

THE COUNTERARGUMENT—SALT IS GOOD FOR YOU

It has been rightly said that salt is the essence of life. The counterargument, that it is wrong to recommend general salt restriction, has two thrusts. The first is that it won't do any good, and the second is that it's downright harmful.

As we saw earlier, changing the salt intake of people with normal blood pressure has, on average, very little effect. But if you look at the individual responses, there are some whose pressure goes down a little, and others in whom it goes up a little. The gadfly doctors who argue that salt restriction is bad have seized on this point, and say that it means that there are some people in whom restricting salt may actually raise their pressure. While it is true that this is theoretically possible, the evidence that this is a meaningful and sustained increase is not there. A much more plausible explanation is that the apparent increase in pressure simply represents random variation: none of us has completely stable blood pressures, which means that sometimes our pressure goes up, and sometimes it goes down.

Another argument is that salt restriction causes the blood cholesterol to go up. There have been a number of studies that show that when people eat a very-low-salt diet, this can happen. It appears to be a temporary phenomenon, however, and is unlikely to be of relevance when eating a moderately low-salt diet. It has also been suggested that if you restrict salt, you're likely to restrict a lot of other important nutrients from your diet. This again is likely to happen only if you go on a really extreme diet, and cut out salt altogether, which no one is seriously advocating. Finally, there is one study that shows that men with high blood pressure who were on a very-low-salt diet at the start of the study, and whose blood pressure was treated with medications during the course of the study, were at increased risk of having a heart attack. While this result is disturbing, no one is sure how to interpret it; for one thing, the men were instructed to eat a low-salt diet on the day on which the evaluation was made. For another, it could be that being on a low-salt diet is not a good thing if you're already taking medications such as diuretics, which themselves cause salt depletion.

The proponents of the "salt is innocent" argument would conclude by saying that the basic tenet of medicine is "first do no harm," and until it is proven beyond all reasonable doubt that restricting salt intake is both effective and harmless, it should not be a universal recommendation.

HOW SALT INTAKE IS MEASURED

Understanding how salt intake is expressed can be confusing, because different units are used to express it. About 40 percent of the weight of a given amount of salt comes from the sodium, and the other 60 percent from the chloride. Salt is usually expressed in grams, 1 teaspoon of salt being about 5 grams. The salt content of foods, however, is given as milligrams (mg) of sodium. Finally, if that isn't confusing enough, salt excretion in the urine is expressed as milliequivalents (mEq). The conversions among these three measures are shown in Table 3.1.

Table 3.1. Conversion of Salt Units

SALT (GRAMS)	SODIUM (MILLIGRAMS)	SODIUM (MEQ)
2.5	1,000	44
5	2,000	88
7.5	3,000	132
10	4,000	176
20	8,000	352

In practical terms, most of the sodium we consume is as sodium chloride, so the conversion table holds up quite well. A typical American diet would be 10 grams of salt per day, or 4,000 mg of sodium, giving a 24-hour urine sodium content of 176 mEq.

HOW MUCH SALT DO WE NEED?

There is no doubt that most of us consume far more salt than we need. This isn't necessarily bad, because our kidneys can normally excrete the surplus in the urine. The amount of salt in our bodies changes very little from day to day despite enormous fluctuations in salt intake. The minimum amount needed to maintain normal bodily functions may be as little as half a gram per day. There are a few situations in which our requirements may be higher than this, such as when we lose salt as a result of diarrhea or sweating during heavy exercise in hot weather, but they are relatively unusual. Very low levels of salt intake, of the order of 1 gram per day, are seen today only in a few primitive societies such as the Yanomano Indians living in Brazil, who are of great interest to blood pressure researchers because they don't develop hypertension. However, there are so many ways in which their lifestyle differs from our own that it's hard to be sure that this is because they don't eat salt.

RECOMMENDATIONS BY PROFESSIONAL AND GOVERNMENT ORGANIZATIONS ABOUT SALT INTAKE

Based on the arguments that I summarized in the previous section, most professional organizations have recommended that salt intake should be moderately restricted if you have high blood pressure. The latest report of the Joint National Committee on the Detection and Treatment of High Blood Pressure has proposed that salt intake be reduced to less than 6 grams of salt (or 2–3 grams of sodium), which for most of us would be a reduction of about one third of our current level of intake. How you can do this is discussed in Chapter 18.

Other organizations such as the American Heart Association have made similar recommendations. Outside the United States, however, the situation is very different. The British Hypertension Society has cautioned hypertensive patients against smoking and heavy alcohol intake, and advised dietary weight reduction, but salt restriction comes at the bottom of the list of priorities. Their recommendation is simply to avoid excessively salty foods. The World Health Organization prescribes weight reduction, restriction of alcohol, exercise, and lastly salt restriction, which was judged to be effective in some patients.

WHAT IS SALT SENSITIVITY?

One of the concepts to evolve over the past few years is that high blood pressure has different mechanisms in different people. A particular type of medication or treatment may work very well in one patient, and not at all in another. Salt restriction is no exception. Studies in hypertensive patients have shown that there is a very wide variation in the extent to which changes in dietary salt intake affect blood pressure. Some people can eat as much or as little salt as they like, without any effect on their blood pressure; they are "salt-insensitive." Others may change their pressure by as much as 5 or 10 mm Hg, and are classified as "salt-sensitive." For some reason their kidneys are not so good at getting rid of the extra salt when they go on a high-salt diet, so their blood pressure goes up. There's no exact definition of salt sensitivity, but a generally acceptable one would be a change of blood pressure of at least 10 mm Hg on going from a high- to a low-salt diet. About 40 percent of people with high blood pressure are salt-sensitive.

HOW DO I KNOW IF I'M SALT-SENSITIVE?

It would be very helpful if there were a simple test that could tell your doctor whether or not you're salt-sensitive. Unfortunately, at the present time there is no reliable method for finding out, other than by systematically trying a period on a low-salt diet, and seeing what happens to the blood pressure. However, the chances of your being salt-sensitive are increased if you

- Are older rather than younger
- Are black rather than white
- Are fat rather than thin
- Are diabetic
- Have a low renin level in your blood

SALT APPETITE—AN ACQUIRED HABIT

Newborn babies do not show any particular craving for salt, but as children grow up they learn to like salty foods, a preference that in most of us persists for the rest of our lives. Nevertheless, people who deliberately go on a low-salt diet may lose the craving, and eventually find very salty foods unpalatable.

SUMMARY

• Salt, technically known as sodium chloride, is a vital component of our bodies. The degree to which eating a high-salt diet raises blood pressure remains controversial.

• The average daily intake of salt in westernized societies is about 7 to 10 grams (or 3–4 grams of sodium). The easiest way to measure salt intake is with a 24-hour urine collection.

• Professional organizations generally recommend reducing salt intake by about one third, to less than 6 grams of salt (2 to 3 grams of sodium).

• People vary greatly in the degree to which restricting salt intake lowers their blood pressure: less than half are "salt-sensitive." In the others (salt-insensitive) it has little effect.

• There is no reliable test for predicting if you're salt-sensitive, although your chances are increased if you're older, black, and overweight.

• A trial of a low-salt diet is certainly worthwhile if you have high blood pressure. The best way to do it is to have your blood pressure and salt intake measured on your normal diet, then go on a low-salt diet for at least a month and have both measurements repeated.

CHAPTER FOUR

HOW YOUR DIET AFFECTS YOUR BLOOD PRESSURE AND YOUR ARTERIES

"You are what you eat" is a common enough saying, and it certainly applies to blood pressure. In this case it's not just what you eat, but also how much, because being overweight is one of the biggest risk factors for developing high blood pressure. Like many other topics discussed in this book, the relationships between diet and blood pressure are complex and still highly controversial. Salt is supposed to be bad for blood pressure, but as we saw in Chapter 3, that's not always the case, and there are many other dietary components that are equally, if not more, important. I will start with a discussion of the major types of food—carbohydrates, fats, and proteins. None of them has a major effect on blood pressure, but fats are of paramount importance in the causation of atherosclerosis. Of greater importance to blood pressure are the minerals. Sodium was discussed in the previous chapter, and here I'll describe the others: potassium, calcium, and magnesium.

An important point about dietary influences on cardiovascular disease is that they are complex: it's not just the intake of one or two constituents that is important, but the whole balance of the diet. This is well illustrated by the conundrum of the French, who eat a high-fat diet but have relatively little heart disease, as described at the end of this chapter.

CARBOHYDRATES—SIMPLE AND COMPLEX

Carbohydrates get their name from the elements from which they are made—carbon, hydrogen, and oxygen. There are two basic forms: the simple carbohydrates, or sugars (sucrose, glucose, and fructose), are relatively small molecules. The complex carbohydrates, or starches, are much bigger molecules, which are made up of large numbers of sugar molecules joined together. Before they can be absorbed into the bloodstream, complex carbohydrates have to be broken down into their component sugars. This is why they take longer to digest than simple carbohydrates. The liver converts other types of sugar into glucose, which is the type used by the body. Not all carbohydrates can be absorbed, however. The indigestible residue is called fiber, which is excreted in the feces. A high-fiber diet is good for all sorts of reasons, which are discussed below.

Virtually all the carbohydrates we eat come from plants. The most notable exception is a sugar called lactose, which is present in milk. Most of us can digest lactose, but there are some people who are "lactose-intolerant," who lack the enzyme needed to do this, and in whom milk products can cause diarrhea and abdominal discomfort.

Contrary to what many people think, carbohydrates are not fattening. An ounce of carbohydrate provides the same number of calories as an ounce of protein, and about half the calories of the same amount of fat.

VEGETABLES AND THE MANY VIRTUES OF FIBER

It is well known that vegetarians tend to have lower blood pressures than meat eaters, and one possible explanation for this is that they eat more fiber, the fad food of the 1980s. The story really started in 1970, when a British physician, Dr. Denis Burkitt, pointed out that many of the diseases common in Western societies, such as cancer of the colon, varicose veins, appendicitis, hemorrhoids, and heart disease, are much less common in regions such as Africa, where fruit and vegetables form the bulk of the diet. He was not actually the first to promote the virtues of fiber. The pioneer here was Dr. John Harvey Kellogg, a Seventh-Day Adventist and vegetarian who, at the end of the last century, ran a sanitarium in Michigan, and who believed in colonic cleanliness. To promote this, he developed numerous nut and vegetable products, and inspired his brother W. K. Kellogg to market cornflakes as a breakfast food. One of the patients at the sanitarium was C. W. Post, who founded the second well-known cereal company.

Fiber is a generic term for complex carbohydrates that come from the cell walls of plants, and is in fact the component of the plant that cannot be digested or absorbed. The most obvious consequence of eating a high-fiber diet is therefore an increase in the bulk of the feces. Fiber thus makes a good antidote to constipation, and has the additional advantage of providing a low-calorie means of filling the stomach.

Fiber is commonly divided into two types—soluble and insoluble. Insoluble fiber comes from the "skeleton" of plant cells, and consists of substances such as cellulose and lignin. Soluble fiber includes sticky substances such as gums and pectins. The two types, and the diseases they are thought to protect against, are shown in Table 4.1.

Table 4.1. Sources and Effects of Soluble and Insoluble Fiber

	SOLUBLE FIBER	INSOLUBLE FIBER
Examples	Pectins	Cellulose
	Gums	Lignin
Sources	Fruits	Vegetables
	Oats, barley	Wheat
	Legumes	Whole grains
	Psyllium	Cereals
Diseases protected against	Hypertension	Colon cancer
	Atherosclerosis	Diverticulosis
	Diabetes	Appendicitis
	Obesity	Hemorrhoids
	Gallstones	Constipation

The effects of fiber on blood pressure have been demonstrated in a recent study conducted by Dr. Keith Eliasson and his colleagues in Sweden. A group of patients with mild hypertension were randomly allocated to receive 20 tablets a day of either fiber or placebo. This amount of fiber corresponded to about half the normal daily intake for Scandinavian populations. After three months of treatment the diastolic blood pressure of the fiber-treated group was 4 mm Hg lower than in the placebo group, although the differences in systolic pressure were not significant. Another interesting result was that the fiber-treated group lost weight, while the placebo group did not. If you have high blood pressure, it thus makes good sense to eat a high-fiber diet.

OTHER REASONS WHY VEGETABLES ARE GOOD

In addition to fiber, vegetables contain a whole host of other substances, whose nutritional benefits are only just beginning to be appreciated. People who eat a lot of vegetables have not only less heart disease but also less cancer. One reason for this may be that they contain antioxidants, a heterogeneous group of chemicals that protect our bodies' cells from being attacked by free radicals, which are discussed in Chapter 24. One such group is the flavonoids, substances with exotic names like quercetin and kaempferol. These occur in a variety of fruits and vegetables, and also tea and wine. A Dutch study found that men whose diets were rich in flavonoids (mainly from tea, onions, and apples) were at reduced risk of getting coronary heart disease.

OAT BRAN

At regular intervals over the past few years, there have been reports of the latest of a series of oat bran studies, with headlines such as "Oat bran found to lower cholesterol," and "Oat bran has no effect on cholesterol." While these statements are clearly conflicting, it's by no means uncommon for medical studies to produce opposite results. The situation has to a large extent been resolved by a recent analysis that looked at all the individual studies and combined the data of the ones that were scientifically acceptable. The conclusion was that oat bran does lower cholesterol, but by only 2 or 3 percent, and to get this result the subjects had to eat 3 grams a day, or one and a third cups of oat bran. A typical serving of cereal would be just under one cup, so that's an awful lot of oat bran. People who had relatively high cholesterol levels to begin with derived more benefit, with a decrease of 6 to 7 percent.

In passing, we may note that attempts to disguise oat bran in forms such as oat bran muffins are a waste of time: they don't actually contain much bran, and any good that it might do is offset by the eggs that are also used in the muffins.

Garlic and Onions

Garlic has a long history of medicinal use, and has been shown to lower cholesterol. Since most people who consume it for medical reasons take it as pills, its effects are discussed in Chapter 24 ("Vitamins and Health Foods"). Onions come from the same plant family as garlic, and their therapeutic effects are the same. An Indian physician, Dr. N. N. Gupta, and his associates studied the effect of including a generous serving of fried onions in men who ate a fatty meal. Four hours after the meal the men who ate the onions had an average cholesterol of 201, while in the others it was 247. The onions also increased the ability of the blood to dissolve clots.

What Are Fats and Triglycerides?

Unless you have taken courses in biochemistry, you're probably confused about the different types of fat, and how these relate to triglycerides. So here's a short chemistry lesson. Ninety-five percent of the fat in our diets consists of triglycerides, which are complex molecules made up of one glycerol molecule joined to three fatty acid molecules (hence the name triglyceride). The fatty acids come in all shapes and sizes, but their common element is that they are all made of a string or chain of carbon atoms of varying length with hydrogen atoms attached to each carbon. The degree of saturation of the fat refers to how many pairs of hydrogen atoms could be added: a saturated fatty acid has no more room for any more hydrogens, while a monounsaturated fatty acid (sometimes abbreviated as MUFA) can accept one pair, and a polyunsaturated acid (or PUFA) more than one (*mono-* is the Greek for one, and *poly-* means many). Saturated fats tend to be semisolid, while unsaturated fats are more liquid, which of course is why they are referred to as oils.

Animal fats are almost all saturated fat, while most vegetable fats are either mono- or polyunsaturated; two notable exceptions are palm oil and coconut oil, both of which are highly saturated. Some of the commoner examples of foods containing the different types of fat are shown in Table 4.2.

Table 4.2. Examples of Different Types of Fats in Commonly Used Foods

SATURATED	MONOUNSATURATED	POLYUNSATURATED
Butter	Avocado	Almonds
Cheese	Cashew nuts	Corn oil
Chocolate	Olive (oil)	Cottonseed oil
Coconut (oil)	Peanut butter	Fish oil
Egg yolk	Peanuts (oil)	Margarine (soft)
Lard		Mayonnaise
Meat		Pecans
Milk		Safflower oil
Palm oil		Soybean oil
Poultry		Sunflower oil
Vegetable shortening		Walnuts

CIS- AND TRANS-FATS: MARGARINE MAY NOT BE THE ANSWER

There is one other variation between different types of fats that we should mention. Unsaturated fats can exist in two slightly different configurations, called *cis-* and *trans-*. The *cis-* form has a kink in the middle of the chain of carbon atoms, while the *trans-* form is straight. The *cis-* forms are liquid, but the *trans-* forms tend to be solid. This difference has been exploited by the manufacturers of commercial vegetable oils. The urge to cut down on the use of saturated fats in cooking has led to an increased use of unsaturated vegetable oils as substitutes. Most of these exist in the *cis-* form, which makes them liquid, and which also limits their utility for some types of cooking. They can be made firmer by a chemical process known as hydrogenation, which changes their configuration into the *trans-* form. Margarine is a major source of *trans-* fats, but it depends on the type: the softer tub margarine contains 17 percent of its fat as *trans-*fat, while the firmer stick form contains 32 percent.

A recent study published in the *New England Journal of Medicine* showed that switching from a diet rich in natural vegetable oils (*cis-*) to hydrogenated oils (*trans-*) raised the LDL cholesterol and lowered the HDL cholesterol, an effect that was just as bad as eating saturated fat. Most of the *trans-*fat in the American diet comes from hydrogenated soybean oil.

There is recent evidence that consuming a lot of *trans*–fatty acids may contribute to the development of heart attacks. A survey of 239 men admitted to hospitals in Boston with a heart attack found that they had a significantly higher intake of *trans*-fats than their healthy counterparts. In men with the highest intake, the risk was increased two and a half times. Supporting evidence in women comes from the Nurses' Health Study, in which 85,000 nurses have been followed since 1980. Women who eat a lot of *trans*–fatty acids, particularly in the form of stick margarine, have a significantly higher risk of having a heart attack than those with a lower level of intake. Interestingly, the same study found no association of heart attacks with the consumption of red meat.

A recent theory proposed by an expert in metabolism, Dr. George Mann, incriminates *trans*–fatty acids as the chief villains in the development of atherosclerosis. Dr. Mann points out that the epidemic of heart disease began in about 1920, a few years after hydrogenated vegetable oils containing *trans*–fatty acids began to be introduced into the American diet. Today, the consumption of *trans*–fatty acids is much higher in northern Europe than in the Mediterranean countries, and the prevalence of heart disease is higher. The French, who eat a high-fat diet but get little heart disease (see "The French Conundrum" near the end of this chapter), also use relatively little *trans*–fatty acids.

These recent findings are somewhat ironic, because many people have switched from butter to margarine on the assumption that they would be less likely to get heart disease. It is also unfortunate that in 1989–1990 the American fast-food industry largely switched from using beef tallow for making French fries to using partially hydrogenated vegetable oils, with a high *trans*–fatty acid content. The studies available to date don't tell us whether it would have been better to have stayed with the butter and the beef tallow, but there are some definite implications: if you are going to eat margarine, choose the tub variety rather than the sticks, and choose natural vegetable oils rather than hydrogenated oils.

GOOD FATS AND BAD FATS

When people talk about fat as a cause of heart disease they usually mean saturated fat, which, as we saw above, includes most types of animal fat. There are a large number of saturated fatty acids (SFAs), which vary according to the number of carbon atoms that make up the chain. Only three of them, with chains of medium length (called lauric, myristic, and palmitic acids), actually raise cholesterol; those with shorter or longer chains have no effect.

The other kind of fat that has been shown to have a bad effect on risk factors for atherosclerosis is hydrogenated vegetable oil, which is described above.

The two other types of fats, polyunsaturated and monounsaturated fats, most of which are of vegetable origin, are also important. From a health point of view, these are good fats, while the saturated fats are the bad fats, because of their different effects on lipids and blood pressure, as shown in Table 4.3.

Table 4.3. Effects of Different Types of Fats on Blood Pressure and Blood Lipids

	LDL CHOLESTEROL	HDL CHOLESTEROL	TRIGLYCERIDES	BLOOD PRESSURE
Saturated fat	↑	—	↑	↑
Hydrogenated oil	↑	↓	↑	
Monounsaturated fat	↓	—	—	↓
Polyunsaturated fat	↓	↓	↓	↓

↑ = increase; ↓ = decrease

The vegetable oil PUFAs (polyunsaturated fatty acids) are also referred to as omega-6 fatty acids, the most important of which is called linoleic acid. Their chief beneficial effect is that they lower LDL (bad) cholesterol, but they may also lower HDL (good) cholesterol. They also inhibit blood clotting.

Fish oil PUFAs are the omega-3 fatty acids, which inhibit the clotting process.

Monounsaturated fats (MUFAs) are found in some vegetable oils and nuts. People who eat a Mediterranean diet rich in olive oil (which contains the MUFA oleic acid) have low cholesterol and little heart disease. As shown in Table 4.3, MUFAs have the most beneficial effects on the blood lipid profile, since they lower LDL cholesterol without adversely affecting HDL (PUFAs tend to lower HDL).

The traditional view is that a diet that is likely to provide the best protection against coronary heart disease is one that has a high quantity of polyunsaturated fats and is low in saturated fats, or, as it's sometimes stated, is a diet with a high P/S ratio.

While there is a lot of support for this idea in general, it's becoming increasingly clear that it's no longer correct. It's now recognized that the amount of monounsaturated fats (MUFAs) in the diet is at least as important as the balance between the saturated (SFA) and polyunsaturated (PUFA) fats. There are at least seven dietary factors that are now recognized as being involved in the process; SFAs and *Trans*-fats promote the development of disease, and the other five help to prevent it. They are listed in Table 4.4.

Table 4.4. Dietary Factors Promoting or Preventing Coronary Heart Disease

PROMOTING FACTORS	PREVENTING FACTORS
Bad fats:	Good fats:
SFAs	Vegetable oil PUFAs
Trans-fats	Fish oil PUFAs
	MUFAs
	Dietary fiber
	Antioxidants

The other two dietary factors that are known to be important are fiber (described above) and antioxidants.

DIETARY FAT AND BLOOD PRESSURE

Seventh-Day Adventists have lower blood pressure than Mormons do. Both religious sects ban the consumption of alcohol, caffeine, and tobacco, but the Adventists are vegetarians while the Mormons are not. Thus the big difference between their diets is that the Adventists eat virtually no fat. They also tend to weigh less, and have less heart disease than the Mormons. The main way in which fat affects blood pressure is that it has nearly twice as many calories per gram as protein or carbohydrate, and, of course, the excess calories are stored in the body as fat. Fat people tend to have higher blood pressures than thin people (the subject of obesity and blood pressure is discussed in Chapter 5).

A large number of studies have investigated the effects on blood pressure of changing the amount and type of fat in the diet. The consensus is that if the total calories are kept the same, not much happens to the blood pressure, so there must be some other explanation for the low blood pressure of vegetarians. The only exception to this statement is fish oil (which is technically a fat), which does lower the pressure when taken in large quantities.

EFFECTS OF A COMBINED LOW-SALT/LOW-FAT DIET ON BLOOD PRESSURE

A few studies have examined the effects of combining salt restriction with a low-fat/high-fiber diet (the type of diet recommended by the American Heart Association, as described in Chapter 18). All have reported that blood pressure was reduced by a significant amount (about 5 mm Hg), and probably to a greater extent than either salt restriction or fat restriction on its own. The fat restriction also tends to lower the blood cholesterol.

NUTS AND HEART DISEASE

Seventh-Day Adventists are a group of particular interest to medical scientists, because they don't smoke, they don't drink, and they usually eat a vegetarian diet. A recent study of more than 31,000 Adventists living in California related their dietary habits to their risk of developing heart attacks. The most striking finding from this study was that people who ate nuts five times a week or more had only half the risk of having a heart attack as those who ate nuts less than once a week. The explanation for this finding is not clear, but it was not just because the people who ate a lot of nuts were vegetarians, and so ate less meat. The authors of the study were not able to say which types of nuts were beneficial, but the ones that the Adventists reported eating were mostly peanuts, almonds, and walnuts.

Although nuts contain a high proportion of fat (which explains why they are also such a rich source of calories), most of it is polyunsaturated fat (the good kind), and they also contain a relatively high proportion of fiber. You might think that eating a lot of nuts would make you fat, but one of the interesting findings of the Adventist study was that the nut eaters were actually thinner than the people who did not eat nuts.

More evidence for the benefits of a nutty diet was provided by a study by Dr. Gene Spiller and colleagues from Palo Alto, California. Participants were asked to supplement their diet with 100 grams per day of almonds. This reduced total cholesterol by 20 mg/dl, without any change in HDL. Total fat intake actually increased, but there was no increase in body weight.

Olé for the Olive

The Greeks, who eat a diet more than 40 percent of whose calories come from fat, have one of the lowest death rates from cardiovascular disease of any westernized country. The solution to this paradox is that virtually all of the fat is in the form of olive oil, of which the main ingredient is the monounsaturated fatty acid (MUFA) oleic acid. The virtues of oleic acid are beginning to be explained. It lowers LDL cholesterol, it may lower blood pressure, and it may even protect LDL cholesterol against oxidation, a process that is thought to be a crucial step in the development of atheroma (see Chapter 2). An interesting study conducted in nine different regions of Italy illustrates these points. A survey of nearly 5,000 men and women found that people who consumed a lot of butter had higher blood pressures and higher blood cholesterol than those whose diet was based on olive oil. A Spanish study compared the effects of three different diets, all of which contained the same overall amount of fat. One of the three diets was rich in saturated fats (equivalent to the typical American diet), one was the Mediterranean diet rich in olive oil (MUFA), and the third was based on safflower oil, and hence rich in PUFA, as recommended by the American Heart Association. The worst was the American diet, which raised total cholesterol and lowered HDL cholesterol. In the middle was the safflower oil diet, which lowered total cholesterol but did not change HDL; and the best was the olive oil diet, which lowered total cholesterol and raised HDL. (In Chapter 18, I advocate adopting the Mediterranean diet rather than the more generally recommended AHA diet.)

There are other reasons why olive oil is beneficial. It's a good source of vitamin E (an antioxidant; see Chapter 24), and it's also good for diabetics. The conventional recommendation for people with diabetes is to eat a low-fat and high-complex-carbohydrate diet, but a diet rich in olive oil results in better control of the diabetes, and a more favorable blood lipid profile, with a higher HDL cholesterol. Finally, there is evidence that Greek and Spanish women who eat a Mediterranean diet high in fruit, vegetables, and olive oil are at reduced risk for breast cancer.

Canola Oil—A Cautionary Note

A form of cooking oil that is strongly advocated by the National Cholesterol Education Program and the American Heart Association as being good for the heart is canola oil. What the recommendations do not tell you is that in 1981 more than 25,000 people living near Madrid in Spain were poisoned by consuming an adulterated form of this oil, from which hundreds died. The history of this phenomenon, which has been officially termed the toxic oil syndrome, makes an interesting and very disturbing story.

You might think that canola oil comes from the canola plant, but in fact there is no such thing. It actually comes from rapeseed, a plant related to mustard, with a bright yellow flower, which is now grown commercially on a large scale, particularly in Canada. Although rapeseed oil in one form or another has been used for cooking for over a thousand years in the Orient, it has been used for this purpose in the Western world for only the past twenty or thirty years. The reasons for its popularity are that it is very low in saturated fat, with a high content of both poly- and monounsaturated fats, and that it is cheap. Despite this apparently "clean" profile, there have been concerns about its safety ever since its introduction that have never been laid to rest. As long ago as 1975 the Swedish Medical Research Council questioned its safety because of experiments in rats showing that it caused degeneration of the heart muscle. This was subsequently attributed to a chemical known as erucic acid, which constitutes nearly 40 percent of native rapeseed oil, and led to the development of strains of rapeseed that produced oil with a lower erucic acid content. The doubts continued, however, and in his Presidential Address for the American Heart Association, Dr. Thomas James warned about the potential dangers to the heart of eating rapeseed oil. Six months later disaster struck in the form of the toxic oil syndrome.

At that time it was illegal to import rapeseed oil as a food substance into Spain, although it could be used as machine oil. To prevent its being used for cooking, aniline, an artificial dye, was added. When the epidemic broke out, a pediatrician named Dr. Tabuenca realized that the common feature of families that were afflicted was that they had bought an adulterated form of rapeseed oil, sold illegally as olive oil by street vendors. The vendors had managed to remove most of the aniline dye, but traces still remained, and the illness was attributed to aniline. The Spanish government offered to replace the adulterated oil with pure olive oil, and the epidemic died out. In 1985 the FDA declared that canola oil "is generally regarded as safe," and the massive marketing campaign in the United States was launched, backed by corporate giants such as Anheuser-Busch and Du Pont. Genetic engineering was undertaken to improve the taste and smell of the oil, which is now widely used in cooking and the preparation of processed foods.

There the story should end, but unfortunately it doesn't. The features of the toxic oil syndrome do not in any way resemble those of aniline poisoning, and can be reproduced experimentally by rapeseed oil, even when it has a low erucic acid content. Despite extensive searches, no other toxin could be identified in the Spanish rapeseed oil. The mystery remains.

In a recent article in a cardiological journal Dr. James concluded with the statement "Whether the growing consumption of rapeseed oil [i.e., canola oil] in the United States proves to be beneficial for the heart, as the NCEP vigorously proposes, or whether it may simply be a way of substituting another and possibly worse form of coronary disease for atherosclerosis, time will tell."

CHOCOLATE—SAFER THAN YOU THINK

There are all sorts of myths about chocolate: it will raise your cholesterol, give you acne, and help you fall in love. The scientific name of the cacao tree from which chocolate is obtained is *Theobroma,* which means food of the gods. One thing that's not a myth is that chocolate contains saturated fats, and hence calories. Although about 50 percent of chocolate is fat, only 1 percent of an average American's daily diet comes from chocolate. In order to set the record straight, the Chocolate Manufacturers of America sponsored a scientific symposium promoting the virtues of chocolate just before Valentine's Day of 1994, which was duly reported in the national press.

The principal fatty acid in chocolate is stearic acid, which is rapidly broken down in the liver to oleic acid, a monounsaturated acid that is also present in olive oil and canola oil. Oleic acid does not raise cholesterol, and a study in which healthy young men were fed a diet rich in chocolate for nearly four weeks confirmed that this was so. So you can enjoy your Valentine's Day gift without feeling guilty.

FISH OIL—THE OMEGA-3 STORY

Omega-3 fatty acids are a group of naturally occurring substances that have been very much in the news lately, having been claimed to be the new panacea, with benefits for a wide variety of chronic human diseases ranging from heart disease to arthritis and cancer. Books on the subject have appeared with names such as *The Omega-3 Breakthrough: The*

Revolutionary, Medically Proven Fish Oil Diet, and health-food stores are full of different types of fish oil capsules marketed by the large pharmaceutical companies, the sales of which now exceed $45 million per year. Since FDA regulations do not apply to such nonprescription medications, many extravagant claims have been made, making one think that fish oil may be akin to snake oil.

The fish oil story started in northwest Greenland, where it was observed many years ago by Danish epidemiologists that Eskimos rarely got heart disease, even though they ate a very-high-fat diet, consisting mainly of whale meat, seal, fish, and seabirds. In fact, the word *Eskimo* is derived from an American Indian word meaning people who eat raw meat. When blood tests taken from Eskimos were compared with tests from Danes it was found that the Eskimos had lower levels of both cholesterol and triglycerides than the Danes, and also that their blood was slower to clot.

It is thought that these differences between the Eskimos and the Danes are due to the large amounts of fish in the Eskimos' diet, and that certain oils in the fish confer protection. The technical name for the class of oils involved is omega-3 polyunsaturated fatty acids (omega-3 PUFAs), and two specific ones are eicosapentanoic acid (EPA) and docosahexanoic acid (DHA). Omega-3s are important because our bodies cannot manufacture them, and because they are the building blocks for a very important class of chemicals called the eicosanoids or prostaglandins, which are involved in all sorts of bodily functions, including the regulation of blood pressure and blood lipids,

They are marketed in health-food stores with names such as Promega and MaxEpa. The main effect of fish oils is to reduce the tendency for blood clots to form, and it has been suggested that they also dilate blood vessels, and hence lower blood pressure. They lower blood triglyceride and total cholesterol levels, and raise HDL.

Studies of the effects of fish oils on blood pressure have given a mixed message. One of the best was conducted by Drs. Howard Knapp and Garret Fitzgerald, who found that high doses of fish oil (50 ml of MaxEpa daily) given over a period of four weeks lowered blood pressure by 6 mm Hg systolic and 4 mm Hg diastolic. A lower dose (10 ml) had no effect. Another study conducted in Norway obtained similar results, but there was no effect of the fish oil supplement in people who were already eating fish three times a week or more. The most extensive was the TOHP (Trial of Hypertension Prevention) study, in which 175 people took 6 capsules (3 grams) per day of Promega; nothing happened to their blood pressure, but some of them experienced an unpleasant taste in their mouth, and belching. A recent review of 31 studies of the effects of fish oil on blood pressure concluded that unless huge doses were taken, the effects were very small.

Other claims have been made for the benefits of fish oils. These include an improvement of symptoms in rheumatoid arthritis, and others that are less well substantiated. There are also potential risks, however. They increase the tendency to bleed, and they may reduce resistance to infections.

The amount of omega-3 fatty acids varies greatly between different types of fish. In general, oily fish (such as trout, salmon, mackerel, and tuna) contain nearly ten times as much as white fish (such as cod, plaice, and haddock).

Fish oil capsules should not be taken in very large doses, because they contain a lot of vitamins A and D, which may be toxic when consumed in large amounts. They also have a lot of cholesterol.

My own recommendation is to eat fish several times per week, particularly the sorts that contain the omega-3 fatty acids, and not to bother with the capsules. This is the same recommendation as made by the American Heart Association.

FISH

Surprisingly little research has been done on the effects of eating fish on blood pressure, although, as we've just seen, there are a lot of studies investigating the effects of fish oils. Dr. Peter Singer in Berlin compared the effects of eating mackerel and herring in 15 healthy volunteers. Mackerel was chosen because it contains a lot of omega-3, while herring has much less. Each diet was eaten as two cans of fish daily for two weeks. The results were quite striking: on the mackerel diet the systolic blood pressure fell by 15 mm Hg, and the diastolic by 7; triglycerides fell by nearly 50 percent, total cholesterol by 7 percent, and there was also an increase in HDL. No consistent changes were seen on the herring diet, although the trends were in the same direction.

It should be remembered that the most important reason for trying to lower blood pressure is to prevent heart attacks, and one of the most convincing arguments for the benefits of eating fish comes from a study called DART (Diet and Reinfarction Trial), conducted on men who were recovering from a heart attack. There were three types of dietary intervention: cutting back on fat, eating more fiber, or eating more fish (at least twice a week). Over the next two years the men in the fish-eating group had one third fewer heart attacks than either of the other groups.

PROTEIN

One of the more unpleasant memories of my early childhood is school lunches in England shortly after the end of World War II. We were told that we did not have to eat all the vegetables, but we had to eat the meat, which was leathery gray slices interspersed with fat and gristle. As every child knew, if you didn't eat meat, you didn't grow.

We're not only older now but also wiser. Most of us eat twice as much protein as we need, and as we grow older, we need even less. If we got all our daily protein from meat, one 2-ounce steak would suffice. (That would be about 60 grams of protein for a 160-pound man.) There's a well-established theory that eating too much protein puts a strain on the kidneys, which have to excrete the excess (unlike fat, protein is not stored if it's not needed). If you have kidney damage from high blood pressure, or if you have kidney disease that's causing high blood pressure (see Chapter 9), your doctor will probably recommend that you eat a low-protein diet.

Another problem with eating lots of protein is that most of it is of animal origin and comes with fat, and that means calories. In a T-bone steak, 20 percent of the calories are from protein; the other 80 percent are from fat. If you trim all the fat off, there will still be 50 percent of the calories from fat. Fish is much better from this point of view: tuna (without oil) has about 60 percent of calories from protein, and white fish such as sole has 90 percent.

You can get all the protein you need from vegetable sources, but you have to eat the right combination to get enough. That's because there are different types of protein. The building blocks from which proteins are made are called amino acids, which contain nitrogen. Our bodies need 22 different kinds of amino acids, most of which we can manufacture, but there are 9 we can't. These are called the essential amino acids, and we have to get them from our diet. The best vegetable source is the bean family (legumes). Examples are tofu (bean curd), lentils, kidney beans, lima beans, and soybeans. Bulgur, which is a grain, is also good. All of these are completely free of fat and salt.

Soy Protein

It is well recognized that there tends to be less heart disease among veg-etarians than meat eaters, and one reason may be that some vegetable proteins can lower blood cholesterol levels. The best example is the pro-tein found in soybeans, whose effects have been the subject of extensive research. An analysis of 38 controlled trials of its effects concluded that an intake of 30 grams or more of soy protein daily could lower LDL cho-lesterol and triglycerides by about 10 percent. This is certainly a sub-stantial reduction, but to achieve it you would need to consume at least three servings of soy protein a day. It's now available in many foods, and you could do it by drinking two glasses of soy milk and eating one serv-ing of tofu—if you think it's worth the sacrifice. You may have trouble finding these foods at your local supermarket, however. You'll come across soy sauce (which doesn't count) and soy burger mix (under names such as Nature's Burgers), but there probably won't be any soy milk in the dairy section. You may do better at a health-food store, where soy protein is sold in products such as tempeh and tofu.

POTASSIUM

While sodium is generally recognized to be bad for blood pressure, there is a lot of evidence that its sister mineral, potassium, may be good. Several studies have shown that giving extra potassium to people with high blood pressure, usually as potassium chloride pills, can lower their blood pressure by a few mm Hg. One of the side effects of diuretics, which are traditionally the first-line drug treatment for hypertension, and which lower blood pressure by depleting the body of sodium, is that they also cause a loss of potassium. It can be argued that the latter may limit their blood-pressure-lowering effect, because if the potassium is replaced, there is a further reduction of the pressure. A recent study conducted at the University of Naples showed that the same effect can be achieved by simply increasing the proportion of potassium-rich foods in the diet. In this particular study the subjects were encouraged to eat more legumes (beans, peas, and lentils), vegetables (potatoes, broccoli, carrots, spinach, and others), and fruit. All the patients in this study were taking medication at the start, but at the end of one year nearly 40 percent of the patients eating the high-potassium diet were able to come off drugs altogether, compared with less than 10 percent in the control group (who continued their usual diet).

Animal experiments have shown that, in addition to lowering blood pressure, potassium may protect against strokes. There's a limited amount of evidence from human studies to support this view. In a study of elderly Californians it has been found that people who consumed more potassium were at lower risk of having a stroke, independently of their blood pressure.

A common custom, which in the light of these findings would seem to make a lot of sense, is to use salt substitutes in which sodium chloride is replaced by potassium chloride (the taste is quite similar). There are dangers with this policy, however. Consuming a large amount of potassium over a short space of time can cause the blood potassium level to rise. In a healthy person the extra potassium is rapidly excreted in the urine, but in older people, who commonly have some impairment of their kidney function, this may not happen, and the high blood potassium can destabilize the heart and occasionally cause a fatal arrhythmia (abnormal heart rhythm). Other situations where excessive consumption of potassium may be dangerous include people who are taking potassium-sparing diuretics, ACE inhibitors, or nonsteroidal antiinflammatory drugs (these are all described in Chapter 22).

CALCIUM

A few years ago calcium was hailed as "the great white healer" in *Prevention* magazine, because of its reportedly beneficial effects on blood pressure and osteoporosis. Since that time, enthusiasm has tempered somewhat, although it's undoubtedly important. Calcium (in the form of calcium carbonate) is the basic ingredient of bones and teeth, and is responsible for much of their physical strength. As we grow older some of the calcium in our bones tends to leach out, making them shrink and become more brittle. The medical term for this is *osteoporosis,* which literally means "porous bones." This process explains why we get shorter as we age, and also why old people are at greater risk of broken bones than younger ones. Osteoporosis is particularly common in women after the menopause, and is accelerated by the associated loss of estrogens. Another factor that contributes to this process is a deficient calcium intake. One reason this occurs is that the consumption of dairy products has been falling in recent years because they are high in fat; but they are also the richest source of calcium in the diet. Calcium absorption is enhanced by vitamin D, which is the reason the vitamin is added to milk.

While getting too little calcium is bad for your health, people who take megadoses of Tums or other calcium-containing antacids can develop kidney damage and other problems. The recommended daily intake is 1,000 milligrams if you're under 65, and 1,500 milligrams if you're older (one Tums tablet has 500 mg).

One of the reasons for thinking that calcium may be of importance to high blood pressure comes from population studies that have examined the association between eating habits and blood pressure. The largest of these is the National Health and Nutrition Examination Survey (NHANES), which collected data on more than 20,000 people across the United States. One of the more unexpected findings to come out of this study was that people with higher blood pressure tended to consume less calcium than those with lower pressure. This study did not show any association between salt intake and blood pressure. Clinical trials that have examined the effects of giving extra calcium to lower blood pressure have been disappointing, however, with the average reductions being very small.

MAGNESIUM

Magnesium is another mineral that is important in maintaining normal bodily function, and it has recently been touted as a possible treatment for high blood pressure. You're probably familiar with magnesium as milk of magnesia, an over-the-counter remedy for constipation. Magnesium is a constituent of bones, and plays a role in the manufacture of proteins and in nerve conduction. The main dietary sources are leafy vegetables, nuts, and grains. Most people probably get too little magnesium rather than too much.

Several studies have investigated whether taking extra magnesium, usually in the form of magnesium chloride pills, will lower blood pressure. The results have mostly been disappointing. The best study, called the Trial of Hypertension Prevention (TOHP), found no effect of six pills a day given for six months to 206 men and women, other than a slight increase in the incidence of diarrhea.

IRON

It has been suggested that one reason women get less heart disease than men is that they tend to be iron-deficient as a result of menstruation, and excessive amounts of iron in the body may accelerate atherosclerosis. This idea was never very popular until a few years ago, when a Finnish study reported that men with high body iron stores were at increased risk of having a heart attack. This story made the front page of *The New York Times,* but subsequent studies in Canada, Iceland, and the United States have failed to confirm it. One possible explanation may be that the high iron levels in the Finns may reflect a high meat intake, and it is the fat in the meat, not the iron, that causes the trouble.

THE FRENCH CONUNDRUM

When the death rates from coronary heart disease in different countries are compared to the levels of fat intake, there is a strong tendency for the rates to be highest in the countries where people eat the most fat. At the head of the list are the Finns, who eat a lot of meat and cheese, and at the bottom are the Japanese, who eat very little. Americans come near the top, but the most striking deviation from this trend are the French, who have the same fat intake as Americans, but only one quarter the death rate from heart disease.

One popular explanation of this conundrum, which first reached the public eye on CBS's *60 Minutes,* is that it is the red wine the French drink that confers the immunity. While it may certainly contribute, it's probably not the whole story. Sabine Artaud-Wild, a nutritionist at the Oregon Health Sciences University, and her colleagues recently compared the diets of the French and the Finns to try to explain the difference. They concluded that there were three important factors in the diets that could account for the different rates of heart disease. The first was that the French ate a lot more vegetables and nuts than the Finns— for example, 30 times as many olives and peanuts and their oils—and the second was that they consumed much less milk and butter. The protective effect of the vegetables could be from the greater amounts of monounsaturated fatty acids and the greater amount of antioxidants. The damaging effect of milk could be from its tendency to make blood clots more likely to occur, as has been shown in animal experiments. The third factor was the greater alcohol (particularly wine) consumption of the French.

Other analyses have pointed out the downside of the French diet: the life expectancy of the French is no longer than in other similar societies, which means they must be dying from other causes, one of which, cirrhosis of the liver, is related to alcohol intake.

This analysis has an important lesson. Most people are aware of the fact that to cut down their risk of heart disease they should eat less fat and cholesterol, but not that eating more vegetables may also be beneficial. The message here is to consider your entire diet, and to maintain a healthy balance.

EAT FAT AND LIVE LONGER—THE GREEK EXPERIENCE

Another population that is even more remarkable than the French, although it has not received nearly as much attention, is the Greeks. They break all the rules, and yet their risk of heart disease is among the lowest of the westernized world. The life expectancy of a 45-year-old Greek man is about two years longer than for an Englishman or American of the same age. Greek men smoke heavily, drink alcohol regularly, rarely indulge in recreational exercise, and eat a high-salt, high-fat diet.

What's the answer to this paradox? The only rational explanation is the nature of the diet. Although it's high in fat, almost all of it is in the form of olive oil, which is, of course, a MUFA (monounsaturated fat—see the earlier section in this chapter, "Good Fats and Bad Fats"). The Greeks cook just about everything in olive oil, and rarely if ever use butter or margarine. They eat little meat (and also little fish), but eat a lot of cheese.

Fortunately for the Greeks, they have not yet read the official and politically correct dietary guidelines of the American Heart Association (see Chapter 18), according to which they should be restricting their fat intake. Unfortunately for the Greeks, they are abandoning their traditional diet as the inevitable invasion of McDonald's and Burger King takes its toll.

The lesson to be learned from the Greeks is that you don't have to go on a low-fat diet to cut your risk of heart disease; what you do need to do is to make sure that the fat you eat is mostly MUFA.

THE HOMOCYSTEINE STORY

Homocysteine is probably not a substance with which you are familiar, but it's one that made headlines in 1995 as a risk factor for heart disease. How it got there makes an interesting story. More than thirty years earlier, a young pathologist at Harvard Medical College, Dr. Kilmer Mc-Cully, was impressed with his finding that children who died from a rare hereditary disease called homocystinuria had the sort of arterial disease that is usually seen in 60- or 70-year-olds. One of the features of this disease is an abnormally high level of an amino acid (amino acids are nitrogen-containing acids from which proteins are made) called homocysteine in the bloodstream. In 1969 Dr. McCully proposed that the homocysteine could damage the arterial wall and promote the development of atherosclerosis. He carried out animal experiments that supported his idea, but nobody took much notice, and he subsequently lost his job at Harvard because he hadn't made a sufficient reputation for himself as a scientist. His work was largely forgotten for many years until recently, when two large epidemiological studies, the Physicians' Health Study and the Framingham Heart Study, both reported that people who had high homocysteine levels in their blood had an increased risk of having atherosclerosis. Other research has shown that about 10 percent of the population inherits an inefficient form of the enzyme that clears homocysteine from the blood. This is different from the defect that causes homocystinuria. Even in people who have the inefficient enzyme, however, the main reason for a high homocysteine level is usually an inadequate intake of folic acid and the B vitamins (B_6 and B_{12}), all of which are found in vegetables. You can get your homocysteine level measured by a blood test, although it's not yet widely available.

The good news is that high homocysteine levels can be lowered by taking extra amounts of folic acid and the B vitamins (described in Chapter 24). However, it remains to be seen if taking extra folic acid can reduce the risk of heart disease.

SUMMARY

• Your diet has a major effect on your blood pressure and also your tendency to develop arterial disease.

• Vegetarians have low blood pressure, little heart disease, and also get less cancer than meat-eaters, so a diet with a lot of vegetables is highly recommended.

• Fats are not all bad for your arteries, although they are all equally rich in calories. Fats do not have much effect on blood pressure.

• Of the three major varieties, the worst are the saturated fats (SFAs), which come from animal fat (but not fish).

• Polyunsaturated fats (PUFAs) are safe, and are found in vegetable oils and fish. Fish also contain omega-3 fatty acids, which are beneficial for preventing heart disease.

• The best sort is the monounsaturated fats (MUFAs), the main sources of which are olive oil and nuts. Olive oil is the basic ingredient of the Mediterranean diet, which is associated with a low prevalence of heart disease.

• Margarine is not a good substitute for butter, even though it contains polyunsaturated fat and no cholesterol. It contains synthetic (*trans-*) fat, which is thought to cause atherosclerosis. Soft (tub) margarine contains less *trans*-fat than the solid (stick) type.

• Potassium helps to lower the blood pressure, and may have other beneficial effects. Fruit and vegetables are good sources.

• Calcium lowers blood pressure little if at all, but is necessary to prevent osteoporosis (weak bones) in older people. Antacid pills and low-fat dairy products are good sources.

CHAPTER FIVE

OBESITY AND BLOOD PRESSURE

If you're overweight, this chapter and Chapter 19 ("Losing Weight") may be the most important ones in this book. Obesity may truly be called an American disease, or if not a disease, at least an obsession. In some people's eyes, unfortunately including many doctors', it denotes an image of not only physical ill health but also a lack of moral fiber—people get fat simply because they indulge themselves. While there is some truth in this assertion, it is by no means the whole story.

Let's start by looking at some of the facts and figures. In a recent Consensus Development Conference organized by the National Institutes of Health, the following statistics were given:

- More than a quarter of Americans are overweight.
- As many as 40 percent of women and 24 percent of men are trying to lose weight at any one time.
- People who enroll in weight-loss programs usually lose about 10 percent of their weight, but two thirds of this is regained after one year, and almost all of it after five years.
- More than $30 billion is spent every year in America on efforts to control obesity.

Being overweight is harmful not only because it's a major cause of high blood pressure, but also because it's associated with other risk factors for cardiovascular disease, as well as several other disorders.

How Is Obesity Defined?

Just as with high blood pressure, there is no hard-and-fast definition of obesity. The conventional definition is based on the relationship between body weight and height, and is expressed as the body mass index (BMI, sometimes referred to as Quetelet's index), which is your weight in kilograms divided by your height in meters. In practice, most people use the tables of ideal body weight adjusted for height. These are given in Chapter 19.

Why Do We Get Fat? The Bottom Line: Energy Intake and Output

The term *fat cat* usually brings to mind the vision of an overweight capitalist whose corporation has a very healthy balance between revenues and expenses in its accounts. The analogy with accounting is actually quite appropriate for understanding obesity. Fat is equivalent to stored energy, and over the long term, what happens to our body weight is determined by the balance between energy intake and expenditure. Fat cells represent the body's investment of surplus energy to tide it over in hard times. Some people could be fatter than others either because they eat more, or because they expend less energy, or both. You might think that it would be relatively easy to decide which of these factors is the most important, but in practice it has been very difficult to get any consensus, partly because energy intake and expenditure are quite difficult to measure accurately, and perhaps also because different factors may be important in different individuals. Many studies have concluded that fat people do not eat more than thin people, which implies that they expend less energy. There are two mechanisms by which the body expends energy. The first is by physical activity, and the second is by metabolism, or the generation of heat. This can be measured as the basal metabolic rate (BMR). Studies of prisoners in Vermont showed that doubling the intake of calories for as long as six months produced very little increase of weight, on average, even though there was no increase in the amount of physical activity. The presumption was, therefore, that the subjects were simply burning up the excess energy by increasing their metabolic rate.

There is a lot of evidence that obesity tends to run in families, but this could be either because it is genetically determined, or because different members of a family tend to adopt the same habits of eating and exercise. An ingenious study conducted by Dr. Albert Stunkard in 540 Danes who were adopted shortly after birth has helped to resolve this question. It was found that whether or not the adoptees were fat was not related to the fatness of their adoptive parents, but was related to the fatness of their true, or biological, parents. The authors of this study concluded that genetic influences were more important than the family environment in determining obesity. In another study 12 pairs of twins were fed an additional 1,000 calories per day for seven weeks. Some of them put on a lot of weight during this time, and others very little. The crucial point was that each member of the twin pairs put on about the same amount of weight as the other. What this study tells us is that, if you overeat (as most of us do), how much weight you will put on lies in your genes.

But what is it that is inherited? Two recent studies have indicated that it may be energy expenditure that is the culprit. In the first, the intake and expenditure of energy of babies born to fat and thin mothers were compared. The babies who put on the most weight during the first year of life were the ones who had the lowest total energy expenditure, mainly as a result of lower physical activity. The second study investigated American Indians from Arizona, a group particularly susceptible to obesity. It was found that the ones who gained the most weight over a two-year follow-up period had the lowest overall energy expenditure at the start of the study. Thus, it appears that people who stay thin burn up their surplus energy, while those less fortunate store it as fat.

A much publicized recent finding has been the discovery of an "obesity gene" which regulates the sensation of hunger in animals. Whether the same gene exists in people is unknown.

These studies should not be interpreted as meaning that your body weight is predestined by your genes, and that you're powerless to change it. They do, however, emphasize the importance of looking at both sides of the energy equation—you need to exercise as well as diet if you're going to lose weight.

The fact that, with the right incentive, it is possible to change your weight in either direction is well illustrated by some recent achievements of movie stars who needed to change their weight in order to play their parts. Indeed, the ability to do this may become a measure of their dedication to their craft, and perhaps also of their Oscar-winning potential. Robert De Niro added 56 pounds to play the part of boxer Jake La Motta in the movie *Raging Bull*. He did this by eating his way through France and the rest of Europe, and as he said at the time: "It's very hard. You've got to get up and eat. Eat that breakfast, eat those pancakes, even if you're not hungry. It's murder." His efforts paid off, and *Raging Bull* was rated the best movie of the eighties by critics. Kathleen Turner, who was criticized as having become too heavy, did the opposite. For her movie *Undercover Blues,* the studio spent $65,000 on slimming her down with a six-week tour of gymnasiums in East Hampton and New York, for a daily regimen of five hours of exercise and an hour of aikido, supervised by her personal trainer. In conjunction with a low-fat diet, this helped her lose a total of 22 pounds. Despite this effort, however, the movie was not a success.

THE FATTENING OF AMERICA

Despite the huge growth of the diet industry (see Chapter 19), Americans are growing fatter. A series of national surveys conducted between 1960 and 1991 has shown that in the past 15 years there has been a dramatic increase in the prevalence of obesity by nearly 10 percent, while in the preceding 15 years it was only 2 percent. Why this should be happening is not altogether clear, but is probably due to a number of factors, including poor dietary habits, more sedentary lifestyles, and quitting smoking. This is particularly worrying, because weight-loss programs are relatively unsuccessful, and prevention is much more effective than treatment.

Even more worrying is the finding of a recent study of 116,000 women who were followed for 14 years, which showed that a weight gain of 11 to 18 pounds after the age of 25 was associated with a 25 percent increase in the chances of having a heart attack. The same thing almost certainly applies to men.

OBESITY AND BLOOD PRESSURE

In just about any society in the world, it has been found that fat people have higher blood pressures than thin people. As we grow older, most of us tend to put on weight and develop middle-age spread. In westernized societies, blood pressure also goes up with age, so it's interesting to note that in societies in which body weight does not typically increase with age, neither does blood pressure. Nevertheless, in spite of this general association between body weight and blood pressure, the actual correlation between them is not very close, meaning that there are a lot of fat people with low pressure, and conversely a lot of thin people with high pressure. On average, if you're 20 pounds above your ideal weight, your blood pressure is likely to be 2 to 3 mm Hg higher than if your weight was normal. The risk of hypertension associated with obesity is particularly strong in younger people: in a large population survey made a few years ago in the United States (known as NHANES, or National Health and Nutrition Examination Survey), the risk of being hypertensive was five times higher in obese people than in thin people aged 20 to 44, but only twice as high in people above the age of 45. In another large survey (the Hypertension Detection and Follow-up Program) it was estimated that 6 out of every 10 hypertensive individuals were more than 20 percent overweight, so in every sense of the word, obesity is a big problem.

Longitudinal studies, in which people are observed over a period of many years, have shown the same thing. In the Framingham Heart Study, men and women who were initially aged between 30 and 62 were followed for 12 years, and it was found that those who were more than 20 percent above their ideal weight at the start of this period were eight times more likely to develop hypertension than those who were 10 percent below their ideal weight. There have also been several studies that have investigated the effects of weight loss on blood pressure. A recent example is the Hypertension Prevention Trial, in which 200 overweight individuals with high-normal blood pressures were started on a weight-reduction program. After six months the average loss of weight was 10 pounds, and the blood pressure fell by 5 mm Hg. Other studies have reported generally similar results.

OTHER REASONS WHY BEING OVERWEIGHT IS BAD

Obesity is bad not only because it raises blood pressure, but for a whole host of other reasons as well. Fat people tend to have higher blood levels of total (mainly bad) cholesterol and also lower levels of HDL (good) cholesterol. Not surprisingly, therefore, they are also at higher risk of developing heart disease.

Diabetes is also much more likely to occur in fat people, particularly the adult-onset variety, for which the risk is increased nearly threefold by obesity.

Gallstones, which are mainly composed of cholesterol, are also commoner in overweight people.

Another metabolic problem associated with obesity is gout, which can cause a very painful type of arthritis. Many people think (wrongly) that taking diuretics (water pills) will help them lose weight, but one of the main side effects of these medications is to bring on an attack of gout.

The commonest form of arthritis (osteoarthritis) occurs because of prolonged wear and tear on the joints, and the more you weigh, the more will be the pressure on your weight-bearing joints. One of my overweight and hypertensive patients has had to have both knees replaced—they simply couldn't take the strain.

More alarmingly, there are several types of cancer that are associated with obesity. In men these include colon and prostate cancer, and in women cancer of the breast, uterus, and gallbladder.

There are also important social consequences of obesity. A survey of adolescents performed in 1981 showed that those who were overweight were less likely to be married 10 years later and more likely to have lower incomes.

THE DEADLY QUARTET, OR INSULIN RESISTANCE SYNDROME (IRS)

Four risk factors for coronary heart disease (obesity, hypertension, high triglycerides, and high blood insulin) often coexist in the same individual, and this combination has been termed "the deadly quartet" or insulin resistance syndrome (a name perhaps more easily remembered by its acronym, IRS). Some of these individuals also have diabetes, of the sort known technically as non-insulin-dependent diabetes mellitus, or NIDDM for short. Diabetes is characterized by a high blood sugar, and insulin lowers blood sugar—for example, by promoting its uptake by muscles, which burn it up during exercise. In the other sort of diabetes, seen in young thin people, there is a deficiency of insulin, but in NIDDM, which occurs in older and overweight people, there is resistance to the effects of insulin (the muscles don't take up the sugar as they should), and insulin levels in the blood are actually increased as part of the body's attempt to overcome this. In this condition the resistance to insulin may be restricted to the muscles, and it is thought that the increased insulin levels may raise the blood pressure, either by causing the kidneys to retain salt or by stimulating the sympathetic nervous system. This excess insulin may also be responsible for the high triglyceride levels, because the liver is still sensitive to the effects of insulin, and converts into fat the excess sugar that the muscles won't take up.

IRS can actually be produced experimentally by feeding rats a typical American diet—high in sugar and in fat.

These points explain why high insulin levels and insulin resistance are bad news. They also explain why the beer-belly or "apple" type of obesity seen predominantly in men is more dangerous than the cellulite or "pear" obesity more characteristic of women, because only apple obesity is associated with insulin resistance.

There is no routine test done to see if you have the IRS, but you don't really need one. If you have the characteristics described above (overweight, high blood pressure, high triglycerides, and low HDL), you almost certainly have it.

The good news is that the condition can be treated quite effectively with a combination of diet and exercise. A study conducted at the Pritikin Longevity Center in California showed that a 26-day boot-camp regimen of a low-fat/low-salt diet, with abstinence from alcohol, caffeine, and nicotine, together with a vigorous exercise program produced substantial reductions in blood levels of insulin, sugar, and triglycerides, and also of body weight and blood pressure. There's a catch, however. If you simply switch from eating fats to eating carbohydrates (by which I mean sugar and starch) without any attempt to cut down on calories, you may actually put on weight, because the surge of sugar in the blood after a heavy pasta meal stimulates the release of insulin, which turns the sugar into fat, and also stimulates your appetite. This subject is discussed further in Chapter 19.

APPLES AND PEARS—BAD FAT AND GOOD FAT

One of the more interesting medical advances of recent years has been the realization that it is not simply the amount of fat in your body that influences your health, but where it is laid down. There are two general types of obesity. The first is the centrally distributed variety that is typical of men, where most of the fat is in the trunk and abdomen, and gives them the apple shape or beer belly. The second is the lower-body (pear-shape) variety affecting the hips and thighs, which is the concern of so many women pumping pedal machines at health clubs.

They are the lucky ones, because study after study has shown that apple fat is worse than pear fat. Which sort you have is measured very easily, by the waist-to-hip ratio. All you need is a tape measure: if your waist girth is greater than your hip girth (both measured at their widest point), your waist-to-hip ratio is greater than one, and you have a problem—you're an apple type. If it's less than one, you may not look terrific on the beach, but otherwise you don't need to worry because you're a pear type.

Increased abdominal fat is associated with a high cholesterol, and a higher mortality from hypertension and heart disease. There's also an increased probability of having diabetes.

The reasons central obesity is so much worse than obesity in the thighs are beginning to be appreciated. Fat deposited in the abdomen is metabolically very active, and is constantly being broken down and reconstituted. These fatty breakdown products get into the circulation and may be deposited in the walls of arteries, as atherosclerotic plaque. A second consequence of the release of fatty acids is that they result in higher levels of insulin circulating in the blood (the liver normally removes much of the insulin secreted by the pancreas, but not when it's soaked in fat). As discussed above, this combination of high fat and high insulin is thought to be particularly bad. In contrast, fat that is deposited in the thighs is metabolically inactive—it just sits there. Where your fat is deposited is dictated by the blood levels of the male hormone testosterone.

Although smokers generally weigh less than nonsmokers, a recent study reported that smoking is associated with a central distribution of fat.

Leptin—The Ultimate Cure for Obesity?

For many years it has been suspected that there is a circulating substance that regulates body weight, because when the circulation of a thin mouse is experimentally hooked up to the circulation of a fat mouse, the fat mouse loses weight. Until very recently, it was impossible to isolate this substance, presumably because it is present in such small amounts. Then Dr. Jeffrey Friedman and his colleagues at Rockefeller University in New York isolated a gene from a strain of obese mice, which they called the ob gene. Genes make proteins, and with modern techniques it is possible to insert a gene into a bacterium to give you a little protein factory. This was done with the ob gene. It led to the production of large amounts of the protein, which was named the OB protein, or leptin. In July 1995 the journal Science published a trio of articles describing the effects of the protein in mice. The message was basically the same in all three: daily injections of the protein caused fat mice to become thin mice in only a few weeks, and without suffering any adverse effects. It even made thin mice become thinner mice, and appeared to work by making the mice both eat less and burn more calories.

Is this the magic bullet we've all been waiting for? Time will tell, and it will be several years before there is a possibility of a drug for human use. Meanwhile, the drug companies are already rubbing their hands with glee: one of them (Amgen) has paid Rockefeller University $20 million for a patent license.

SUMMARY

• Obesity is a national obsession: more than a quarter of Americans are overweight, and a third are trying to lose weight, mostly without success. And as a nation, we're getting fatter.

• People get fat for two reasons: excess intake of calories and insufficient expenditure of energy. The latter is determined partly genetically (by your basal metabolic rate) and partly by your level of physical activity.

• Obesity is associated with high blood pressure: for every 10 pounds you put on (or lose), your pressure is likely to go up (or down) by 5 mm Hg.

• Other reasons that obesity is bad for your health include an increased risk of diabetes, heart disease, gallstones, arthritis, and some types of cancer.

• The distribution of body fat is also important. The central or "beer-belly" obesity characteristic of men is more closely linked to cardiovascular disease than the lower-body obesity seen in women.

• A common combination of risk factors is the "deadly quartet"— high blood pressure, central obesity, latent diabetes (insulin resistance), and high triglycerides. It can be treated with diet and exercise.

CHAPTER SIX

PHYSICAL INACTIVITY AND BLOOD PRESSURE

One of the less attractive features of modern civilization is the fact that we eat too much and exercise too little. The recently introduced and derogatory term "couch potato," describing someone who sits in front of a television set eating potato chips, is also a perfect description of an individual at risk of developing high blood pressure and heart disease. Less than 20 percent of Americans exercise to a level needed to achieve physical conditioning and cardiovascular benefit, and 40 percent are sedentary. A recent survey of more than 2,000 ten-year-old American girls found that one of the best predictors of how fat they were was the number of hours each day they spent watching television.

The benefits of regular exercise are well illustrated by a recent survey conducted in young adults (ages 18 to 42) living in Tecumseh, Michigan, a typical rural midwest community. Seventy percent said that they took no regular exercise. Compared with the fitter 30 percent, they weighed more and had higher blood pressures, higher total cholesterol and triglyceride levels, and lower HDL cholesterol. There were also psychological consequences, such as more anxiety, more anger, and a greater feeling of time pressure. The benefits of exercise were apparent even in people who exercised only once a week.

LACK OF EXERCISE AS A RISK FACTOR FOR HIGH BLOOD PRESSURE

The evidence that physical inactivity is a risk factor for hypertension is compelling. Numerous population surveys have shown that people who say they exercise regularly have lower blood pressure than those who say they don't, but there's a catch here, because such people also tend to weigh less. A more convincing study has been carried out by Dr. Ralph Paffenbarger (a sage exercise advocate who runs 50-mile ultramarathons) in Harvard alumni. One of the reasons for studying this particular group is that Harvard, like other colleges, is heavily dependent on its alumni for financial support, and consequently has a very efficient organization for tracking their whereabouts and state of health. In his study he followed the progress of 15,000 alumni for 6 to 10 years, and found that men who exercised regularly were less likely to become hypertensive than men who did not. This could not be accounted for by any differences in body weight.

LACK OF EXERCISE AS A RISK FACTOR FOR HEART DISEASE

One of the themes of this book is that blood pressure is important only to the degree to which it predisposes people to strokes, heart attacks, and other forms of cardiovascular disease. Several of the benefits of exercise relate to the prevention of heart disease rather than to the reduction of blood pressure. A good example of this comes from a study known as the Lipid Research Clinics Mortality Follow-up Study, which was designed to evaluate the role of cholesterol in causing heart disease, but also collected information about physical fitness, which was measured by having the subjects perform an exercise test. There were 4,276 men tested, and they were divided into four groups according to their level of fitness. The men in the fittest group tended to have lower blood pressures and lower cholesterol levels. Over the next eight and a half years the rate of death from cardiovascular disease was eight times higher in the least fit group than in the most fit.

There are also numerous studies that show that people who exercise regularly are at lower risk of developing coronary heart disease than those who do not. In a survey of 18,000 British civil servants who all had sedentary jobs, Dr. Jeremy Morris and his colleagues found that those people who reported that they had indulged in some form of physical exercise during the previous weekend had half the risk of having a heart attack over the next eight years as those who said that they had not exercised. Similar findings were reported by Dr. Paffenbarger in his study of Harvard alumni: those who exercised regularly were at lower risk than those who were sedentary. It's also clear that the exercise doesn't have to be leisure-time activity. Dr. Paffenbarger followed 6,000

San Francisco longshoremen over a 22-year period. The men who had physically active jobs had half the risk of heart disease as their colleagues whose jobs were sedentary. He also found that the protective effect of exercise was lost after four years of stopping exercise.

The explanation for the beneficial effect of exercise is most probably its impact on the traditional risk factors for heart disease. This was the conclusion of a study from the Honolulu Heart Program, which followed 8,000 men living in Hawaii for 23 years. Those who exercised regularly were at 25 percent less risk of dying from coronary heart disease, and this reduction in risk could be accounted for by the finding that these men had less obesity, less hypertension, less diabetes, and lower blood cholesterol than the sedentary men.

BLOOD PRESSURE CHANGES DURING STATIC AND DYNAMIC EXERCISE

In Chapter 1 we saw how the brain can regulate the blood pressure to meet the different needs of the body, such as occur during static and dynamic exercise. Static exercise is defined as a sustained contraction of a muscle group, and is typified by weight lifting. Dynamic exercise is characterized by intermittent and rhythmical contractions; examples are running, bicycling, and swimming. The effects of these two types of exercise on blood pressure are different: during static exercise there is a marked increase of both systolic and diastolic pressure, whereas with dynamic exercise only the systolic pressure increases. Many activities involve a mixture of both types of exercise: walking with a heavy suitcase is one example. The effects of different types of exercise on blood pressure are well illustrated by a study that investigated the effects of hammering in different positions. Hammering nails into the floor produced a relatively small increase in blood pressure, while hammering them into a wall raised it more. By far the biggest increases occurred when the nails were being hammered into the ceiling, however. This may be explained on the grounds that the awkward position needed in the latter situation involved sustained contraction of some muscle groups, which was what made the blood pressure go up.

BLOOD PRESSURE CHANGES AFTER EXERCISE— POSTEXERCISE HYPOTENSION

Immediately after a prolonged bout of exercise the blood pressure falls to levels below its resting value. This can occur after any type of exercise that uses large muscle groups, such as walking, running, bicycling, and swimming. The lowest level is seen at about 30 minutes after the end of the exercise, and may be as much as 20 mm Hg (systolic) below the resting level. Over the next three to four hours it gradually returns to baseline.

This fall in blood pressure occurs in virtually everybody, particularly after more prolonged periods of exercise (20 minutes or longer), but the changes are more pronounced in people with higher blood pressures—the pressure falls more, and stays down longer, sometimes as much as 12 hours. So if you have high blood pressure yourself, that's good news.

The degree to which this phenomenon contributes to the effect of exercise training on resting blood pressure is not known at present, but we can presume that the two are connected. We also don't yet know whether your blood pressure will be lower at work if you've exercised that morning than if you haven't, but we anticipate that it might be.

THE MEASUREMENT OF PHYSICAL FITNESS

When we talk of someone being in good shape, or physically fit, we generally imply that he or she exercises regularly. While exercise habits and fitness are obviously related, the two are not the same. According to the President's Council on Sports and Physical Fitness, physical fitness means "the ability to carry out daily tasks with vigor and alertness without undue fatigue, with ample energy to enjoy leisure time pursuits and to meet unforeseen emergencies." It thus encompasses a number of factors, such as cardiovascular conditioning, body composition, flexibility, and muscle strength. It is usually measured by how well one does on a standard exercise test, using either a treadmill or a stationary bicycle. Some of us are better athletes than others, and two people who have trained to the same degree will not necessarily do equally well on the treadmill test.

The most accurate measure of aerobic fitness is the maximal oxygen uptake, which is how much oxygen your body can burn during exercise. This is somewhat cumbersome to measure in practice, and since during dynamic exercise oxygen consumption and heart rate are very closely related, for most purposes the measurement of heart rate and blood pressure at different levels of exercise is sufficient. The other commonly used index of fitness is the length of time that one can keep going on a treadmill.

Although maximal oxygen uptake is not routinely measured, there is evidence that if you exercise enough to get a conditioning effect and increase your maximal uptake, your cardiovascular risk is reduced to a lower level than with more moderate exercise.

EFFECTS OF EXERCISE TRAINING ON BLOOD PRESSURE

It may seem paradoxical that exercise raises blood pressure acutely, and yet lowers it over the long term, but there are now numerous studies that demonstrate this. Typically, the procedure is to take a group of hypertensive subjects who at the start of the study are untrained, and to put them through a training program lasting for several weeks. Most studies have found that this results in a gradual reduction in the resting level of blood pressure of about 5 mm Hg.

EFFECTS OF EXERCISE TRAINING ON BLOOD LIPIDS

An analysis of 66 exercise studies that examined the effects of training on blood cholesterol concluded that the changes occurring in the average subject who exercised regularly were as shown in Table 6.1.

Table 6.1. Effects of Regular Exercise on Blood Lipids

Total cholesterol	Decrease of 10 mg/dl
LDL cholesterol	Decrease of 5 mg/dl
HDL cholesterol	Increase of 1 mg/dl
Triglycerides	Decrease of 16 mg/dl
TC/HDL ratio	Decrease of 0.5

Note that these are all changes that should cut your risk of heart disease. The changes are not the same in everyone, of course. One factor that seems to determine the extent of the changes is what happens to body weight: if this goes down, the chances are that the lipids will also improve, but if it goes up, the lipids are likely to get worse also. You may have to exercise quite a lot to have much effect on the HDL cholesterol, perhaps the equivalent of walking or running 8 to 10 miles a week.

EXERCISE TRAINING AND AGING

Most of the risk factors for heart disease, including blood pressure, tend to get worse as we age. A lot of this is related to "middle-age spread." Most of us tend to consume more calories than we expend, and the surplus gets stored as body fat. These trends were well demonstrated in the Healthy Women Study currently being conducted at the University of Pittsburgh. Five hundred women in their forties were followed over a three-year period. They had their cardiovascular risk factors evaluated at the beginning and end of the study, and were also asked about their exercise habits. The average increase of blood pressure was about 1 mm Hg, but the total and LDL cholesterol went up by 10 mg/dl, the HDL went down 1 mg/dl, and the weight increased by 5 pounds. The women who were most physically active showed the smallest weight gain, and were also less likely to have a decrease of their HDL cholesterol. Another benefit of exercise was a lower probability of depression.

We don't normally recommend weight-lifting programs to 87-year-olds, but that's exactly what Dr. Maria Fiatarone and her colleagues at the Hebrew Rehabilitation Center in Roslindale, Massachusetts, did, with dramatic results. A group of nursing home residents took part in a vigorous exercise program, and improved their muscle strength by 100 percent, their walking speed by 10 percent, and their ability to climb stairs by 25 percent. You're never too old to exercise!

SUMMARY

• Lack of exercise is a risk factor for developing high blood pressure and heart disease.

• Both systolic and diastolic pressure increase during static (weight-lifting) exercise, but only systolic increases during aerobic exercise, which may be followed by a period of low blood pressure lasting several hours.

• A program of regular exercise has numerous benefits. They include weight loss, lower blood pressure, lower cholesterol levels, lower risk of heart disease, and a delay in some of the effects of aging.

CHAPTER SEVEN

SMOKING, ALCOHOL, AND CAFFEINE

One of the more depressing features of books giving medical advice is that they tell you to give up doing many of the things you most enjoy. As someone once said, even if you follow the advice, there's no guarantee that you'll live any longer—it will just seem like it. Alcohol, caffeine, and smoking have all been condemned by purists, but as we'll see, smoking is the only unequivocal villain.

SMOKING

The effects of smoking have been likened to the plague in the Middle Ages. In the United States it is estimated to be responsible for nearly 350,000 deaths each year, 225,000 of which are from heart disease, and most of the rest from cancer. Together with high blood pressure and high cholesterol, smoking is one of the Big Three risk factors for coronary heart disease. Each risk factor results in an approximate doubling of risk when present, but because there are more people who smoke than have high blood pressure or cholesterol, smoking accounts for more deaths than either of the other two. In my practice I often see patients who have a particularly virulent form of arterial disease, with manifestations of blockages in the arteries supplying their heart, brain, kidney, and legs. Virtually all of them are smokers.

Chemicals in the tar of tobacco smoke injure the delicate lining of the arteries and make them more susceptible to the deposition of atheromatous plaque. The nicotine in tobacco smoke also contributes to the damage. It's a powerful stimulant, and via its effects on the brain and nervous system activates the nerves regulating the heart and blood vessels, resulting in an increase in heart rate, constriction of the arteries, and an increase in blood pressure. Smoking is also associated with an increase of total and LDL cholesterol (the bad sorts), and a decrease of HDL (the good sort).

THE POLITICS OF SMOKING

In an op-ed piece in *The New York Times* entitled "Alarm Clocks Can Kill You. Have a Smoke," Dr. Elizabeth Whelan, who is the president of the American Council on Science and Health, described how popular women's magazines frequently run articles on health issues, ranging from the hazards of the lead covers on wine bottles to the electromagnetic fields emanating from alarm clocks—issues that most of us would regard as trivial. One health issue that such magazines never discuss, and which accounts for a nontrivial 350,000 deaths a year, is smoking. The explanation for this paradox lies in the magazines' advertising pages, which are full of ads for cigarettes, portraying their users as glamorous, feminine, and above all, thin. And the reason why the United States has a lower cigarette tax than almost any other Western country is not hard to find, either: politicians rely on massive contributions from tobacco manufacturers to help finance their campaigns.

The situation is changing, however, and the tobacco companies are on the run, at any rate in the United States. The bans on smoking in workplaces are extending to locations such as McDonald's restaurants, baseball stadiums, and transatlantic flights. The chief of the Food and Drug Administration, Dr. David Kessler, has told a congressional hearing that he believes that nicotine is an addictive drug and should be regulated as such. He also accused the tobacco companies of systematically manipulating the nicotine levels of cigarettes in a manner reminiscent of Tom Lehrer's song "The Old Drug Peddler":

"He gives the kids free samples, because he knows full well
That today's young innocent faces will be tomorrow's clientele."

At the same hearings the chiefs of the major tobacco companies testified with disarming ingenuousness that they did not believe that smoking causes cancer, and thereby identified themselves as the modern equivalent of flat-earthers. Two scientists who had been employed by Philip Morris reported that their research had shown that nicotine was as addictive as cocaine, and that their findings had allegedly been suppressed by the corporation.

SMOKING AND HIGH BLOOD PRESSURE

Although it has been known for many years that smoking a cigarette raises the blood pressure, it used to be assumed that this effect was only transient, because numerous epidemiological studies have found that people with hypertension are no more likely to be smokers than those with normal blood pressure. One possible explanation for this might be that smokers tend to weigh less than nonsmokers, and the effects of obesity and smoking on blood pressure cancel each other out. But even when smokers and nonsmokers of the same body weight are compared their blood pressures are the same. In our research, we thought that this might be because when people have their blood pressure checked in a doctor's office they usually haven't just smoked, so we compared the blood pressure of smokers and nonsmokers using ambulatory blood pressure monitoring, which enables us to record blood pressure for 24 hours while people go about their normal activities (see Chapter 16). What we found was very interesting: even though the smokers' blood pressure was no different from nonsmokers' in the clinic, during the daytime the smokers' pressures were on average 5–10 mm Hg higher than the nonsmokers'. During the night there was once again no difference. To be classified as a smoker for this study, the subjects had to smoke at least one pack a day, and we interpreted our findings as showing that this amount of smoking can cause a sustained elevation of pressure throughout the day, and that the effects wear off during the night.

SMOKING AND BODY WEIGHT

It is a well-established fact that smokers tend to be less fat than nonsmokers, and when they quit smoking they tend to gain weight. This, of course, is one reason why people go on smoking, and how Virginia Slims got their name. Smokers don't eat less than nonsmokers, and they don't exercise more. The explanation for the slimming effect of smoking is that nicotine directly increases the body's metabolic rate, so more energy is burned up. This effect is enhanced during physical activity.

WHY PEOPLE SMOKE

Ask any smokers why they smoke, and you'll get the same answer: they like it. Nicotine has a stimulating effect on the brain, and produces a complex array of psychological changes. Its effects are apparent within a few seconds of taking a puff. By changing puffing behavior, the smoker can control the dose of the drug to produce its optimal effects. Cigarette smoking is a convenient and socially acceptable way of administering to oneself hundreds of doses of a psychoactive drug (approximately 200 shots per day for someone who smokes one pack of cigarettes per day). It reduces the level of anxiety, which is why people find it helpful during stressful experiences. It has also been shown to enhance people's adaptation to unpleasant stimuli. Unlike tranquilizers, however, it can actually improve one's ability to concentrate and to perform complex mental tasks. Although it attenuates the subjective feelings of stress, it actually augments the bodily response. Both mental stress and smoking a cigarette raise heart rate and blood pressure, and when they are combined the changes are even bigger.

What keeps the tobacco companies in business, however, is the addictive nature of nicotine. In a recent survey 91 percent of Americans said they thought that smoking was an addiction, and they are correct. This subject is reviewed in more detail in Chapter 20.

PASSIVE SMOKING

Over the past few years there has been increasing concern about the effects of passive smoking (or environmental tobacco smoke, as it's referred to in scientific articles). If you're sitting in a waiting room next to someone who's smoking, your heart rate and blood pressure are likely to go up, and there will be a measurable decrease in the oxygen-carrying ability of your blood. Nine out of 10 large surveys concluded that people who don't smoke themselves, but live with a smoker, have a risk of heart disease that is higher by about 30 percent than it would be otherwise. It has been estimated that this could account for 37,000 deaths from coronary heart disease each year.

Will My Risk Go Down If I Quit?

Everything that you've read so far about smoking is bad news, but the good news is that if you can give it up your risk will go down. This statement is based on the findings of several studies. One such, which was conducted by Dr. Lynn Rosenberg at the Boston University School of Medicine, compared the risks of heart attacks in men who were current smokers with one group of men who had quit for less than two years, and with another who had quit for longer than that. For the current smokers the risk was nearly three times higher than in nonsmokers; for those who had quit for less than two years it was down to twice normal, and for those who had not smoked for more than two years it was the same as if they had never smoked.

ALCOHOL

The relationship between alcohol use and heart disease has been much in the news lately, culminating with the claim that drinking red wine helps to keep your arteries clean. Appropriately, it was also the French who first reported that heavy drinking can raise blood pressure. In 1915 a Dr. Lian observed that soldiers in the French army who drank more than 3 liters of wine a day had an increased likelihood of having high blood pressure. Incidentally, 3 liters is more than most people's intake of any fluid in one day! Since that time, numerous epidemiological studies have confirmed this association, although with much more temperate intakes of alcohol. The relationship between alcohol intake and blood pressure may not be a simple one, however. Many U.S. studies have shown that the blood pressure of people who drink small amounts of alcohol (one or two drinks a day) may be a little lower than the pressure of nondrinkers. However, people who have three or more drinks per day have a systolic pressure that is 3–4 mm Hg higher than nondrinkers' and a diastolic pressure 1–2 mm Hg higher. With five or more drinks per day the systolic pressure is typically 5–6 mm Hg higher than in nondrinkers, and the diastolic 2–4 mm Hg higher. Many of the studies that showed these associations between alcohol use and blood pressure were unable to show any influence of salt intake on blood pressure.

EFFECTS OF ABSTAINING ON BLOOD PRESSURE

It has also been clearly established that people who change their drinking habits are likely to show parallel changes in blood pressure. This has been observed in the Framingham Heart Study, for example, where it was reported that an increased consumption over four years was associated with an increase in blood pressure, while a decreased consumption lowered the pressure. This is not just because of changes in body weight; it seems to be from a more direct effect of alcohol on blood pressure.

One of the first experimental studies of the effects of alcohol withdrawal on blood pressure was carried out by Dr. John Potter and Dr. Gareth Beevers in Birmingham, England. They studied 16 moderately hypertensive men who consumed 6 to 8 drinks per day, and found that when alcohol was withdrawn, the blood pressure plummeted by 13/5 (systolic/diastolic) mm Hg within four days. When drinking was resumed, the pressure went back up.

Another important study was conducted by Dr. Lawrence Beilin and his colleagues in Perth, Australia. They recruited 59 men with hypertension being treated with medication, who were all regular drinkers (mostly of beer, since this was Australia). Subjects were randomized either to continue their regular drinking or to reduce their intake to the equivalent of less than one alcoholic drink per day, by switching to low-alcohol beer. Within each group, half were allocated to a low-salt diet, and half to a regular-salt diet. The interesting finding in this study was that restricting alcohol lowered blood pressure significantly (by 5/4 mm Hg), while restricting salt did not. Furthermore, the combined effects of salt and alcohol restriction were no greater than the effect of alcohol restriction alone. This study provides another demonstration that alcohol intake influences blood pressure more than salt intake does.

RED WINE AND HEART DISEASE

There has been a lot of publicity recently about the fact that the French eat a relatively high-fat diet, and yet have much less heart disease than Americans. It has been suggested that this may be because they drink a lot of alcohol, and that red wine may protect them from heart disease. There may be a constituent of wine that reduces the stickiness of blood platelets, and hence the tendency for blood to clot. There is almost certainly more to it than that. In Chapter 4, I discuss this "French Conundrum," and an analysis showing that two other factors may be that the

French also eat more vegetables and drink less milk than other national-
ities with similar fat intakes. This same analysis, which looked at the
heart disease rates and diets in 40 different countries, also concluded
that in Mediterranean countries where the fat intake is very low (for example, Greece and Portugal) the rate of heart disease is low regardless
of the level of alcohol intake. But in countries where the fat intake is
high (for example, France and Finland) a higher alcohol intake was associated with less heart disease.

CAFFEINE: STORM IN A COFFEE CUP

No subject arouses more controversy than the association between coffee and heart disease. Some experts regard coffee as a dangerous drug
that can raise blood pressure, raise cholesterol, and accelerate the development of coronary heart disease, while others consider it to be
harmless. The question is clearly an important one, if only for the stag-
gering size of the numbers involved. Here are some of them:

- Coffee is the major agricultural import in the United States, and is
  second only to oil.
- More than half the U.S. population drinks at least three cups of coffee per day.
- In the past 30 years, consumption of caffeinated coffee has halved,
  but consumption of decaffeinated coffee has nearly quadrupled.
- Americans drink 139 billion cups of coffee a year, of which 20 percent is decaffeinated coffee.

THE EFFECTS OF COFFEE ON BLOOD PRESSURE

Numerous studies have shown that drinking one or two cups of coffee
raises the blood pressure by about 5 mm Hg, which occurs because of
constriction of the arteries. These effects are smaller in people who
drink coffee regularly, suggesting that the effects may wear off with
time.

Large-scale epidemiological studies, in which the blood pressures of
coffee drinkers have been compared with nondrinkers', have given
rather inconsistent results. The best method of resolving whether coffee
drinking has any sustained effects on blood pressure is to carry out a sys-

tematic study of the effects of abstinence. Two such studies are particularly noteworthy. Drs. Annette Bask and Diederick Grobbee in Holland recruited 107 young healthy coffee drinkers, and allocated them into three groups: one continued to drink filtered coffee, one switched to boiled coffee, and one stopped drinking coffee altogether. At the end of nine weeks the blood pressure was 3/4 (systolic/diastolic) mm Hg lower in the group that had stopped drinking, but was unchanged in the other two. In the second study Dr. Robert Superko and his colleagues allocated 150 coffee-drinking volunteers to three groups. One continued to drink coffee, one switched to decaffeinated coffee, and the third quit drinking coffee. Blood pressure was evaluated not only by the traditional clinic measurements, but also by ambulatory monitoring (this technique is described in Chapter 16). In this case there were no changes in clinic pressure, but the average blood pressure measured over the whole day by the ambulatory monitor fell by 3/2 (systolic/diastolic) mm Hg in the subjects who either switched to decaffeinated coffee or quit altogether.

Drinking coffee can also exacerbate the blood-pressure-raising effect of other stressors. When taken with a cigarette, the blood pressure may increase by more than 10 mm Hg over the next hour or two, and coffee also exaggerates the response to mental stress.

COFFEE AND BLOOD LIPIDS

The evidence concerning the effects of coffee on cholesterol and other blood lipids is no less confusing. Many epidemiological studies, particularly from Scandinavia, have found slightly higher levels of cholesterol in coffee drinkers, but more recent investigations have indicated the effects depend on how the coffee is brewed. Scandinavians make their coffee by boiling the ground beans with water, and it has been found that the higher cholesterol levels are mainly seen in people who drink boiled coffee, and not in those, such as most Americans, who drink filtered coffee. Since the caffeine content is equally high whether the coffee is boiled or filtered, this led to the idea that there is something else that might be the culprit. In an experiment that may hold the record for the amount of coffee brewed at any one time, a Dutch nutritionist named Peter Zock boiled 300 pounds of coffee with 2,400 pints of water, and then extracted from the brew a residue that was rich in coffee oils but had relatively little caffeine. He then fed this brew to volunteers for several weeks and observed a progressive rise in blood cholesterol and triglycerides.

In the same study in which the effects of coffee drinking on blood pressure were investigated, Dr. Robert Superko examined the changes in blood lipids. Giving up coffee by itself had absolutely no effect, whereas switching to decaffeinated coffee raised the LDL cholesterol without affecting HDL or triglycerides. But another very similar study (by Dr. Roy Fried) got quite opposite results. He found that drinking filtered coffee raised both HDL and LDL cholesterol, while decaffeinated coffee had no effect. Even here, however, the overall effects of coffee were not necessarily bad, since the adverse effect of the higher LDL would be offset by the beneficial effect of the higher HDL.

On balance, therefore, it appears that if you drink filtered coffee, as most of us do, the effects on your blood lipids will be minimal.

THE BOTTOM LINE—DOES COFFEE DRINKING CAUSE HEART DISEASE?

In the light of this inconsistent information about the effects of coffee drinking on the risk factors for cardiovascular disease, the logical next step is to examine its associations with coronary heart disease itself. It will by now come as no surprise to you to learn that here again the experts are in disagreement. The most definitive analysis of the evidence was recently provided by Drs. Martin Myers and Antoni Basinski. Dr. Myers, a Canadian physician, was concerned that the Canadian Health and Welfare Report had stated that drinking more than four cups of coffee a day would increase the risk of coronary heart disease. (The American Joint National Commission had made no such judgment.) Their analysis examined 11 large prospective studies, 6 of which were done in the United States, 4 in Scandinavia, and 1 in Japanese Hawaiians, with a grand total of 143,030 individuals, most of whom were men. When the results of these studies were pooled, the risks of developing coronary heart disease during the period of observation (which ranged from 2 to 35 years) were exactly the same whether or not the subjects drank coffee. This finding held even in people who drank as much as six cups a day. Of particular interest was the finding that 3 of the 4 studies performed in Scandinavia (where, as we have seen above, the custom of drinking boiled coffee seems to raise cholesterol) found no adverse effect of drinking coffee on heart disease.

WHAT ABOUT DECAFFEINATED COFFEE?

On the grounds that there is no conclusive evidence that coffee is a risk factor for coronary heart disease, there seems to be no reason to advise coffee drinkers to switch to decaffeinated coffee as a means of lowering the risk of a heart attack. There may, of course, be other reasons. One thing that caffeine does do is to cause palpitations (skipped beats) in some people, and if you experience these, it may be worth switching to decaffeinated coffee. If coffee does raise blood cholesterol, it is quite likely that this effect is due to something other than the caffeine. Most decaffeinated coffee is made from a different variety of coffee bean than the one used for regular coffee, and it is possible that there may be more of this cholesterol-raising substance in this other variety.

IF I HAVE HIGH BLOOD PRESSURE AND DRINK COFFEE, SHOULD I QUIT?

The balance of scientific evidence relating coffee drinking to heart disease indicates that if there is any connection, it is very weak. While the counsel of perfection might be to advise patients with high blood pressure or otherwise at risk for heart disease to stop drinking coffee (as is done, for example, at the Pritikin Centers), it seems to me that it is more appropriate to focus on risk factors about which we are more certain. It is hard enough to persuade people to stop smoking, lose weight, and eat less saturated fat, so let's not get too concerned about coffee.

A NOTE ON TEA

Coffee and tea are often lumped together as if they were interchangeable, but they are not. Both are drunk in large amounts, and both contain caffeine, but there the similarity ends. Tea contains antioxidants called flavonoids, and a Dutch study found that men who drink a lot of tea are at reduced risk of heart disease. The same study found no beneficial effect of drinking coffee. It's also possible that tea may protect against cancer.

SUMMARY

• Smoking is bad for many reasons: it is a major risk factor for heart disease, stroke, and lung cancer. It also raises blood pressure.

• Smoking is a chemical addiction as strong as other drug addictions.

• The good news about smoking is that your increased risk of heart disease is reversible if you quit.

• Drinking alcohol raises blood pressure: each extra daily drink raises the pressure by about 1 mm Hg.

• Despite this, moderate drinkers (two drinks a day) have less heart disease than abstainers. This is probably because alcohol also has a beneficial effect on blood lipids.

• Don't worry about coffee; there's no good evidence that it's a risk factor for cardiovascular disease.

CHAPTER EIGHT

STRESS AND BLOOD PRESSURE

Most patients think that stress plays a major role in their hypertension; most doctors do not. Stress management techniques have become very popular for treating it, but as we'll see, their effectiveness in holding down blood pressure is questionable. *Stress* is a rather vague term: we all know what we mean by it, but we're hard put to give it an exact definition. As Humpty-Dumpty said to Alice in *Through the Looking Glass*, "When I use a word it means just what I choose it to mean—neither more nor less." In general, we can regard stress as an individual's perception of an unpleasant or threatening situation over which he or she has little control. This could include a whole variety of things, ranging from physical stress (such as pain) to mental stress (such as a hectic job). An important point to emphasize is that it is a very personal or subjective experience: while there are many things that we all consider stressful (war, for example), there are others that may be acutely stressful for one individual but not for another. Speaking in public might be one such example. In other words, stress, like beauty, is in the eye of the beholder.

How Our Bodies React to Stress

How you respond to stress depends on a number of factors: the nature of the stressor, how stressful you perceive it to be, and also how your body reacts to it. Much of the research that has been done on stress and blood pressure has focused on this last factor, which is referred to as reactivity. The way it's evaluated is by sitting a person in a laboratory and measuring a variety of body functions both while the individual is resting peacefully and while he or she is exposed to stressful situations, each of which typically lasts for five minutes or less. These often include physical stressors, such as putting one hand into ice water, and mental stressors, such as doing mental arithmetic or mirror drawing. This type of research has shown that there are considerable differences among different individuals in blood pressure responses to such stimuli. Men tend to be more reactive than women. This, however, may have more to do with how men and women perceive the different challenges than with anything innate: an ingenious study conducted by Marianne Frankenhaeuser, a Swedish psychologist who is one of the pioneers of stress research, showed that when confronted with a crying child, women are more reactive than men. Dr. Robert Eliot, an American cardiologist and stress researcher, has coined the term *hot reactor* to describe people who show an exaggerated blood pressure response, and has proposed that they are at increased risk of getting high blood pressure and heart attacks. It's an attractive idea (unless you're a hot reactor yourself), but at the moment it's not much more than that. We simply don't know what the long-term implications are of being a hot reactor.

Many years ago, Dr. Caroline Bedell Thomas, a physician at Johns Hopkins Hospital in Baltimore, started a prospective study of medical students to see what factors would predict which ones would develop high blood pressure in later life. One of the most important predictors was whether or not their parents had high blood pressure, but Dr. Thomas also had the students do a reactivity test known as the cold pressor test, in which the blood pressure response to putting one hand into ice water was measured. These individuals have now been followed for more than 20 years, and some of them now have high blood pressure. Her own analysis concluded that the hot reactors were not at increased risk, but a later analysis came to the opposite conclusion. Several other studies have used the same test to predict hypertension, but most have found that it's not of much use. Even if it is found that such a test does predict who's going to develop high blood pressure, it doesn't necessarily mean that stress is contributing to the process. Scientifically speaking, all we can say is that a particular test may be a predictor, but we don't know why. The supposition is that the response to one kind of stress (in this case the iced water) predicts the response to the stresses of everyday life, but this is unproven.

The Effects of the Stresses of Everyday Life on Blood Pressure

A more fruitful approach than studying the effects of simulated stress in the laboratory may be to see what happens to blood pressure during the real stresses of daily life. Until recently, it was very difficult to do this, but with the development of ambulatory blood pressure monitoring it's now quite easy. People can go about their normal daily activities while a miniature device takes readings of their blood pressure every few minutes. Every time a reading is taken, they are asked to write down in a diary what they were doing and feeling. Studies using this technique have shown that both physical and mental activity raise the blood pressure. Talking on the telephone, for example, can put it up by 5 mm Hg. When you're relaxing or watching television the pressure goes down by about the same amount.

Our own research has shown that in most people the blood pressure is highest when they're at work or commuting. What happens when you get home in the evening depends on who you are: If you're a woman it usually goes down if you're single, but if you're married and have children it's likely to stay high. If you're a man it usually goes down whether or not you have children. Our explanation for this finding is that women with young children who work during the day are exposed to two sources of stress—from their job during the day and from their family duties during the evening. The findings in men are not very complimentary to the male sex.

While these types of studies have provided a lot of very interesting information about the normal pattern of blood pressure responses to the stresses of everyday life, they don't necessarily tell us whether such stresses are contributing to the development of sustained hypertension. There is, for example, no evidence to date that women who have a full-time job while bringing up children are at increased risk of hypertension, or any other disorder, for that matter.

Can Stress Produce Sustained Hypertension?

The idea that stress can contribute to the development of hypertension has been around for many years, but there's surprisingly little agreement among the experts as to how important it is. Scientific proof of any relationship involves being able to measure the relevant factors, and one of the problems with stress is that it is very hard to measure it in any objective way. Furthermore, hypertension is a creeping condition that takes many years to develop: if my blood pressure increases at an annual rate that is half a millimeter of mercury greater than yours, after ten years I may be classified as being hypertensive, while you will still be normotensive. And proving that my life has been more stressful than yours over this same ten-year period is obviously not going to be easy. While I may have had some stressful episodes, they are likely to have been of different types at different times, and different from the sorts of stresses to which you have been exposed.

Despite these problems there are a number of studies that lend support to the idea that stress can have long-term effects on blood pressure. A good example is a study of Italian nuns, whose blood pressures were compared with the pressures of women of the same age living in the outside world. The nuns' blood pressures showed little tendency to increase with age, in contrast to the other women's. This could not be explained by any differences in body weight or diet, and was attributed to the nuns' cloistered lifestyle.

Anthropologists have long been interested in primitive societies, many of which show no tendency for blood pressure to increase with age, as it does in modern societies. One example is the bushmen of the Kalahari in southern Africa, who lead (or led) a nomadic life of the traditional hunter-gatherer, and whose blood pressure remained low as they aged. But when they abandoned their traditional ways and became farm laborers, their pressure went up by about 15 mm Hg. Another very similar example is the Samburo tribesmen of Kenya, who were nomadic warriors. When they joined the Kenyan army, their blood pressure also increased. Dr. Ingrid Waldron and her associates reviewed 84 similar studies of the effects of acculturation and concluded that higher blood pressures were associated with increasing emphasis on a market economy, increased economic competition, and decreased family ties.

The interpretation of such findings has been that there is more stability in the social structure of such traditional societies than in our own: they all know their place, and they are not threatened with losing their jobs. A tribe is like an extended family, and this feeling of togetherness is lost when the tribesman leaves to seek his fortune in a big city. While this explanation sounds plausible, it is not the only one. The transition to a westernized lifestyle is usually accompanied by the adoption of a westernized diet, which contains more salt and more calories than the traditional diet. An alternative explanation, therefore, is that it is the diet that is responsible for the increase of blood pressure, and not the stress. This point was demonstrated very nicely in a study of another Kenyan tribe, the Luo, in whom measurements were made of blood pressure, body weight, and salt intake over a period of two years, during which time some of the tribesmen stayed in the villages, while others migrated to Nairobi. The blood pressure of the migrants increased within one month of moving, and they also ate more salt and put on weight. Over the next two years, the migrants' blood pressure stayed up, but the weight gain did not persist. The authors of the study suggested that the stress of migration had resulted in a retention of salt and water by the kidneys, which would explain both the rapid weight gain and the rise of blood pressure.

THE DEFENSE AND DEFEAT REACTIONS

The *defense reaction,* a term used to describe the physiological response to challenges in the natural environment, was first studied by Walter Cannon, who was a professor of physiology at Harvard in the 1920s. He referred to it as a "fight-or-flight" reaction, because it prepared the individual for a period of intense physical activity, when fighting or fleeing from an aggressor. We all recognize this reaction very well: We become aware of our heart beating faster and stronger, we're afraid, and we start to sweat. Our blood pressure also goes up, in readiness for having to pump blood through the contracting muscles. The flow of blood is altered, with an increased amount going to the muscles, and since the muscles will need glucose in order to keep working, the adrenal glands secrete epinephrine (adrenaline), which releases glucose into the blood from the liver stores.

This reaction is entirely appropriate when the challenge we face is a physical one, as, for example, an athletic competition, and it explains why football players may have sugar in their urine just before a game. But when the challenge is an angry boss demanding an explanation for something we've done wrong, readiness for intense physical activity is (usually!) the last thing we need. Some years ago Dr. J. V. Neel proposed the idea that some chronic diseases (of which diabetes and hypertension would be two examples) could be regarded as "diseases of civilization," and occurred because physiological responses that were adaptive in primitive societies, when the challenges were mainly physical, became maladaptive in modern societies, when the challenges are mostly behavioral. On the evolutionary principle of natural selection, or "survival of the fittest," one might suppose that those individuals who had a better-developed defense reaction would have a survival advantage when threatened with physical challenges from the environment. According to this theory, repeated elicitation of the defense reaction, when it is not followed by physical exertion, could eventually produce high blood pressure. Support for this view was provided by an observation made by Dr. Jan Brod, that in many young patients with hypertension the blood pressure was high, not because their arteries were constricted (the pattern seen in older patients), but because their hearts were pumping more blood, with much of the excess going to the muscles: in other words, even while resting quietly, they showed many of the changes seen during the defense reaction.

A less clearly defined response pattern has been termed the *defeat reaction*. In this case the individual perceives that there is nothing that can be done to overcome the threat, and simply "gives up." There is no readiness for physical activity, and the blood pressure does not go up, although the adrenal glands release a hormone called cortisol, which is secreted during any kind of stress.

Dr. Jim Henry spent many years studying experimentally induced hypertension in mice, and has used these two reactions to explain the changes he observed. The mice were housed in a system of cages designed to promote social interaction and conflict. Each cage was a box big enough to hold a few mice, and was connected to other cages by narrow tubes, wide enough only to let one mouse through at a time. When mice were reared in this system, a social hierarchy developed, with some animals becoming dominant and others subordinate. Interestingly, high blood pressure developed in the dominants, but not in the subordinates. Actually, the highest pressures of all were seen in the subdominants striving to achieve control, whose pressure was higher than in dominants whose position at the top of the social heap was unchallenged. Henry found that the dominants had high epinephrine levels characteristic of the defense reaction, while the subordinates had high cortisol levels characteristic of the defeat reaction.

Not surprisingly, it has not been possible to replicate these experiments in people, although there are some interesting parallels. A study done on male prisoners found that men living in single-occupancy cells, where there was little opportunity for social interaction, had lower blood pressure than men living in a dormitory. And when men were transferred from a cell to a dormitory, their blood pressure went up. No attempt was made to classify the individuals as dominant or submissive, however.

Is There a Particular Type of Personality Associated with High Blood Pressure?

If people behaved like mice, we might expect that individuals with dominant personalities would be more likely to be hypertensive than the more mousy submissive types. In practice, it's not that simple. Psychiatrists and psychologists have been arguing for fifty years whether there is a "hypertensive personality" and still can't agree. Part of the problem is that personality is a very difficult thing to measure scientifically; the way it's usually done is to give people a series of questionnaires asking them how they perceive themselves and how they would react in certain situations. While these are easily standardized, they have the disadvantage of being based on how individuals see themselves, not how other people see them. The other method is to give them a more or less standardized interview, which is rated by a trained interviewer. This is the method usually adopted for rating the "type A behavior pattern," which is the best-known personality profile that has been associated with a disease process.

When hypertensive and normotensive individuals are compared on their personality profiles, the picture that emerges is confusing. Many studies have found that hypertensives tend to suppress or bottle up their anger and to be more submissive, not more dominant, than normotensives. Other studies, however, have found no differences. The theory that has been proposed is that the hypertensives' anger finds its outlet by being channeled through the sympathetic nervous system, hence raising the blood pressure.

Researchers have also looked to see if hypertensives are more likely to have type A personalities. The concept of type A has changed somewhat over the years since it was first put forward by Meyer Friedman and Ray Rosenman in 1955. They originally described it as a chronic and excessive struggle to achieve too many things in too short a period of time. The type A individual was characterized as being aggressive, ambitious, and hard-driving—in other words, the ideal corporate executive! Most experts now think that the most important component of it is a "cynical hostility," which is not the same as the repressed anger that some people have associated with hypertension. The type A personality has been linked to the development of coronary heart disease, but most studies have not found any connection with high blood pressure.

JOB STRAIN AND BLOOD PRESSURE

For many people today their jobs are a major source of stress, and this is reflected by the finding that blood pressure tends to be highest during the hours of work. The conventional view of a stressful job situation is the harried executive who has to make important decisions. There is increasing evidence, however, to indicate that this view may not be the most appropriate. Research originating in Sweden has developed a concept of stress that has two components, known as demand and control. Demand refers to the intensity of the job, or workload, and control is the amount of decision latitude that you have over your work. By asking a lot of people a series of questions designed to get at the relative degrees of demand and control associated with their jobs, it is possible to construct a grid or "map" of different occupations. According to this model of stress, if you're in control it's less stressful than if you're not, and the jobs that are most stressful, the so-called high-strain jobs, are the ones characterized by high demands and low control. On this basis our harried executive, who's supposed to be in control, should have a less stressful job than someone lower down the ladder. Interestingly, the majority of high-strain jobs are blue-collar rather than white-collar jobs. A typical example is an assembly-line worker, whose rate of working is dictated by the speed of the line, over which he or she has no control. The stressfulness of this type of work was nowhere better depicted than in Charlie Chaplin's classic movie *Modern Times*. This type of work is by no means a thing of the past, however, as illustrated by a recent article in *The New York Times*, describing the life of a Detroit factory worker:

> Fifty-six times an hour, nine and a half hours a day, six days a week—including Saturdays—he installs the rear windshield washer hose and attaches front and rear bumpers, using a special screwgun that makes it easy on his arms and back to tighten screws. He has less than 90 seconds to do it and if he loses his rhythm he falls behind.

Other examples of high-strain jobs are short-order cooks and telephone switchboard operators.

The evidence that a high-strain job may be bad for your health is incomplete but gradually accumulating. Several studies have shown that blue-collar workers are at higher risk of developing heart disease than white-collar workers, and this can't be explained solely by their smoking and dietary habits. It's also well established that if your education stopped at the high school level, you're more likely to become hypertensive than if you went to college. And several studies have shown that workers in high-strain jobs are at increased risk of having heart attacks compared with those in less stressful jobs. Finally, in a study we have performed in 300 men working in different jobs in New York City, we have found that men in high-strain jobs are more likely to be hypertensive. Our analysis of this study, which is still going on, indicates that it takes many years for the hypertension to develop. In men without job strain the pressure changes little over the years, but in the ones with high-strain jobs there is a progressive increase.

So far, we have not found the same thing in women, even though they are more likely to have high-strain jobs. Perhaps they are more resilient to the effects of occupational stress than men, and pay more attention to what is going on at home.

LIFESTYLE INCONGRUITY AND BLOOD PRESSURE

A different approach to describing the relationship between stress and high blood pressure has been adopted by Dr. William Dressler, who coined the term *lifestyle incongruity,* which he defines as the extent to which one's lifestyle exceeds one's financial means. It's measured by evaluating income and occupational status, on the one hand, and possession of material goods, on the other. In a series of studies, Dressler has found an association between lifestyle incongruity and blood pressure.

Dr. Sherman James has invented a related concept that he has called "John Henryism," named after the American folk hero. An individual who scores high on the John Henryism scale is one who believes that he can control environmental stressors through a combination of hard work and determination. James's studies, which have been conducted in blacks in the southern United States, have shown that the struggle for control which John Henryism embodies is related to blood pressure. Thus in one study he found that men whose education was limited and who scored high on John Henryism had higher pressures than men who scored equally high on John Henryism but were better educated. And in another study men who had managed to get good jobs and had high John Henryism scores had higher pressures than those with similar jobs but low John Henryism scores.

Although these two concepts may at first sight appear to be rather different, there is a similar central theme, which can be stated as follows: if you're content with your status in life you're likely to have lower blood pressure than if you're continually striving to improve it.

SUMMARY

• There's no doubt that stress can produce a transient increase of blood pressure; it's less certain whether it raises pressure over the long term.

• High blood pressure is a by-product of a westernized urban lifestyle.

• The factor that contributes to the increase of blood pressure may be a chronic misfit between the individual and the environment; an example of this (in men particularly) is job strain, which means having a demanding job with little control over what you are doing.

• There is no particular personality type associated with high blood pressure.

CHAPTER NINE

WHEN THINGS GO WRONG— STROKES AND HEART ATTACKS

Many people think that cancer is the biggest cause of death in the United States today, but actually it doesn't even come close. Heart disease is way out in front, even though its rate has been declining markedly over the past twenty years. High blood pressure is a major risk factor for both strokes and heart attacks, and treating it reduces these risks, but unfortunately does not eliminate them altogether. The risk of getting a stroke is cut in half, but the risk of a heart attack by only 15 percent.

CORONARY ARTERY DISEASE

The heart muscle, the most important muscle in your body, is fueled by the coronary arteries, which originate in the aorta where it leaves the heart. There are two main arteries, one on the right and one on the left. The right coronary artery supplies the right side of the heart and the lower part of the left ventricle, which is the high-pressure chamber that pumps the blood through our body. The artery on the left divides into two branches (the left anterior descending and the circumflex arteries), which together supply the rest of the left ventricle. These three arteries run down over the surface of the heart, and send branches into the muscle. It's the narrowing or blockage of these arteries by atheromatous plaque that causes coronary artery disease (also known as coronary heart disease).

ANGINA PECTORIS

If you're lucky, the first indication that you have coronary artery disease is *angina,* which is a Latin word for pain; *pectoris* means in the chest. It happens because the heart muscle is becoming starved of oxygen, or is becoming ischemic, as it's known technically. This usually happens during exercise or emotional arousal, and occurs because when you're exercising or angry your heart starts pumping more blood, and hence needs more oxygen to keep it going. The typical description of angina is a tight feeling in the middle of the chest, which comes on during exercise and goes away during rest. Sometimes it goes down one or both arms, or into the neck. In more severe cases it can start during the night, or while you're at rest. In the vast majority of cases it signifies a partial obstruction to one or more coronary arteries, although occasionally it occurs because an artery goes into spasm.

When angina comes on, and the heart is not getting enough blood, there's a telltale change in the electrocardiogram that clinches the diagnosis. This change forms the basis of the stress test, which is performed by walking on a treadmill while the electrocardiogram is recorded. Sometimes the heart may become ischemic without your feeling any pain; this is called silent ischemia, and may show up on the cardiogram.

How Angina Is Treated

The first line of treatment of angina is with medications. These can do two things: they may dilate the coronary arteries so that more blood can get through the narrowed part (in which case they are called vasodilators), or they may stop the heart working so hard, so that it needs less oxygen. Nitrates, of which nitroglycerin is the best-known example, are vasodilators, and so are the calcium-channel blockers. In general, medications that are vasodilators will also tend to lower blood pressure, which explains why some of the medications used to treat angina are the same as the ones used to treat high blood pressure. However, because the coronary arteries behave somewhat differently from arteries elsewhere in the body, not all the medications are equally effective in both conditions: nitrates are not very good for lowering blood pressure, and ACE (angiotensin converting enzyme) inhibitors don't help angina.

Beta blockers are the other mainstay in the treatment of angina. The way they work is by lessening the increase of heart rate and blood pressure that occur during exercise, so that the heart doesn't have to work so hard and uses less oxygen.

If the medications don't control the angina by themselves, or if testing indicates that the coronary artery disease is quite extensive, it may be necessary to relieve the obstruction, with either a bypass operation or an angioplasty.

Coronary Artery Bypass Surgery. This is now the standard treatment for patients who have extensive coronary artery disease, and in some circles, the scar on your chest from your triple bypass can be worn with the same pride as a war wound. The idea of the operation is quite simple; the blocked part of the artery is bypassed by inserting a graft into the artery beyond the block. This is usually done by taking a section of vein from the leg (the saphenous vein, which is the large vein running up the inside of the leg from the ankle to the thigh) and sewing one end into the aorta, and the other into the coronary artery beyond the blockage. Another way of doing it is to use an artery running down the inside of the chest wall (the internal mammary artery).

There are two basic reasons for recommending this operation: one is to relieve angina, and the other (and more important) is that it may improve your life expectancy. The pain from angina can usually be controlled by other forms of treatment, and whether surgery will make you live longer depends on how severe the disease is. If there are major narrowings in all three coronary arteries, or if you did really badly on the stress test, you'll probably live longer if you have surgery. But if you have only one or two narrowings you generally don't need it.

Coronary Angioplasty. This is a relatively new technique, and its role is still controversial. It's performed by passing a catheter (plastic tube) through the narrowed part of the artery, and stretching it open by inflating a sausage-shaped balloon on the end of the catheter (this is the same procedure that's done in the renal arteries, as described in Chapter 14). It may be the best form of treatment for people who have a major blockage of one coronary artery, but is less well suited to dealing with multiple narrowings. The procedure has received a lot of attention from the media, because of recent high-tech developments such as lasers and atherectomy devices. At one time one of the major New York hospitals was running radio commercials advising patients to go and get their arteries cleaned out by laser treatment. These techniques are still very much in the developmental stages, however (and the radio commercials have since come down to earth). The laser device has a laser on the tip of the catheter, which is supposed to vaporize the plaque. The atherectomy devices work on a "Roto-Rooter" principal, and slice out the plaque, which can then be sucked out of the catheter.

The main problem with all of these techniques is that the beneficial effects are often only temporary. One thing they all have in common is that they traumatize the delicate inner lining of the arterial wall, which, as described in Chapter 2, is one of the factors that led to the development of plaque in the first place. The artery reacts to this by forming scar tissue, so that in some cases (about 30 percent) the narrowing may have returned within a few months of the procedure (this is referred to as restenosis).

Unstable Angina

In some patients angina may persist for many years, in which case it's called stable angina, but if it suddenly starts to get worse, and the pain starts to develop while you're at rest, it's called unstable angina. This is a medical emergency, because it may be the overture to a major heart attack.

HEART ATTACK (MYOCARDIAL INFARCTION)

This is the "big one" and occurs when one of the coronary arteries becomes completely plugged. What happens is that a plaque ruptures, exposing a bare area of tissue, which promotes the formation of a blood clot. The blood flow through the artery is completely stopped, so that the muscle it supplies gets no oxygen. The pain that results from this not only is more severe than the pain of angina, but also lasts longer, for hours rather than minutes.

The amount of damage caused depends on where the blockage occurs, and whether there are other arteries supplying the affected muscle. More muscle will be damaged if the block occurs at the origin of the artery than if it's in a minor branch. If the disease has developed gradually over many years and led to minor blockages, neighboring arteries (called collaterals) will open up to supply the ischemic muscle. So when a major blockage occurs the effects won't be so devastating.

The technical name for a heart attack is *myocardial infarction.* Myocardium means heart muscle, and infarction means death of tissue because of a lack of blood supply. The affected muscle cells die, and are eventually replaced by scar tissue. This has two effects: it weakens the heart's ability to pump, but it can also lead to an electrical instability of the heart, by setting up a short circuit in the wiring. This interference with the normal clocklike rhythm of the heart is called an arrhythmia, and may take many forms. Many of us experience skipped or premature heartbeats, which we have all our lives and are quite harmless. The most dangerous form, which can happen after a heart attack, is called ventricular fibrillation. Instead of proceeding through the heart muscle in an orderly fashion, the electrical impulses become chaotic, and the heart muscle quivers all over, but stops pumping. This process explains why some people who have a heart attack simply drop dead, and also why emergency resuscitation can be effective, because an electrical shock administered to the chest may be able to kick the heart back into its normal rhythm.

The important thing if you're having a heart attack is to get to the hospital right away. There are two reasons for this: first, the potentially lethal arrhythmias tend to occur in the first hour or two after the onset of symptoms, and second, it's possible to dissolve the clot that's blocking the artery with medications. This, however, can be done only in the first few hours, because after this the affected muscle will already have died.

Treatment of Heart Attacks

A heart attack constitutes a medical emergency, and as such requires admission to hospital. If the diagnosis is confirmed, and it's within a few hours of the onset of symptoms, medication is given to dissolve the clot that's blocking the artery. These medications are called thrombolytic agents, the most commonly used being streptokinase or tissue plasminogen activator (Activase). Beta blockers are also used, to reduce the strain on the heart.

After you've recovered from a heart attack you're still at some risk of a recurrence, although this risk decreases progressively with time. Several large-scale clinical trials have shown that taking beta blockers for one to three years after a heart attack can reduce the subsequent mortality by about a quarter—a significant benefit. Interestingly, the same has not been found for calcium-channel blockers. If the damage to the heart was sufficiently extensive to weaken its pumping ability, recent studies have shown that the ACE inhibitors (which like beta blockers and calcium-channel blockers are also used for treating high blood pressure—see Chapter 22) can also significantly reduce mortality.

STROKE

A lot of people with high blood pressure are afraid that when they get a headache they are about to have a stroke. Fortunately, they're nearly always wrong. A stroke can occur in two different ways. The first is the same as in a heart attack, when an artery gets blocked by a ruptured plaque or by a bit of plaque that breaks off and gets carried up into the head, where it plugs a small artery. The other is when a vessel bursts, and blood leaks into the brain. The first sort is called a cerebral thrombosis, and the second a cerebral hemorrhage. Headache is the first symptom of a cerebral hemorrhage, but it differs from the usual type of headache in that it comes on very suddenly (like being hit on the head), and because it's followed by symptoms localized to one side of the body. We have a right and a left brain, each of which has its own blood supply, and each of which controls one side of our body.

The symptoms of a stroke depend on which part of the brain is affected. The commonest are weakness on one side of the body (resulting from damage to the area controlling body movement) and loss of speech (from damage to the speech area).

TRANSIENT ISCHEMIC ATTACKS (TIAs)

Usually the damage caused by a stroke is permanent, but in some cases the symptoms may last for less than 24 hours. These are known technically as transient ischemic attacks (or TIAs, for short), and they have a somewhat different mechanism from a major stroke. The carotid arteries, which are the major arteries in the neck supplying the brain, are favorite sites for the development of atherosclerotic plaque. This can sometimes be detected on the routine physical examination by listening over the neck with a stethoscope for the sound of turbulence (bruit) of blood flowing through the narrowed part of the artery. It can also be seen on ultrasound scans of the artery. What happens in a TIA is that a bit of plaque, or a clump of blood platelets sticking to the plaque, breaks off and gets carried up the artery until it lodges in a small branch. Sometimes this may be the artery that supplies the eye, in which case the symptom would be loss of vision in one eye; in other cases it may cause paralysis of an arm or a leg. Fortunately the blockage is usually not per-manent, because the fragment of plaque breaks up further, and gets washed away.

The important thing about TIAs is that they may be the early warning signs of a major stroke. They can be to a large extent prevented by as-pirin and another platelet-inhibiting agent called ticlopidine.

KIDNEY PROBLEMS

The kidneys are afflicted by the ravages of high blood pressure, but un-like the brain and heart, they suffer in silence. Their function is to cleanse the blood of waste products, which is achieved by filtering out the waste products as urine. The functional units are called nephrons, each of which is shaped like a long-tailed sperm. There are about one million in a normal kidney. The head of the nephron, called the glomerulus, is a filter through which the blood is passed into the renal tubule, or tail of the nephron. Most of the filtrate is reabsorbed through the tubules, but what's left passes out of the tail end of the nephron as urine.

As we age we all lose nephrons, but this process is accelerated by high blood pressure, which damages both the arterioles feeding blood to them and the delicate lining of the glomerulus. This subtle but relent-less damage is rarely enough to cause kidney failure requiring dialysis unless the hypertension is really severe.

There is another mechanism by which kidney failure can occur. As we've seen, hypertension accelerates the formation of atheromatous plaque, and this can occur in the renal arteries as elsewhere. If the plaque is large enough to impair the blood flow through the renal artery, it can not only lead to a reduction in renal function, but also cause the blood pressure to go even higher, by a process called renovascular hy-pertension, described in Chapter 14.

SUMMARY

• Coronary heart disease is the leading cause of death in the United States.

• Angina may be the first manifestation of heart disease, and oc-curs when there is narrowing without complete blockade of a coro-nary artery. It can be treated with medication, angioplasty, or bypass surgery.

• A heart attack occurs when an artery suddenly becomes completely blocked by a blood clot. If treated early, it may be possible to dissolve the clot.

• A stroke can occur because an artery supplying the brain either gets blocked or bursts. The resulting brain damage may manifest itself as weakness of one side of the body.

• A transient ischemic attack (TIA) is a ministroke caused by a temporary blockage that gets washed away, with disappearance of the symptoms.

• Kidney damage is another consequence of high blood pressure, but usually produces no symptoms.

CHAPTER TEN

WHITE-COAT HYPERTENSION

For many people who have been told that they have high blood pressure, visiting their doctor to have it checked may be a major source of anxiety. Some of my patients, who have been seeing me for many years, tell me that they can feel themselves tensing up just before their visit, and a few are even aware of sweating and palpitations. When I take their blood pressure and find that it's high, it only serves to reinforce their sense of apprehension.

The observation that the blood pressure recorded by a doctor tends to be higher than when measured in other situations is nothing new. In a classic article published in 1940, Drs. David Ayman and Archie Goldshine taught a group of their hypertensive patients how to monitor their own blood pressures, which they did for periods of up to six months. In many cases the pressures recorded by the patients were as much as 30 or 40 mm Hg lower than the pressures recorded by the doctors. Although these findings were quite dramatic, no one knew what to make of them, because all the information we have about high blood pressure and its consequences is based on measurements made by doctors, not by patients. Nevertheless, the very important question remains: Are the high pressures recorded in the doctor's office more representative of the patient's "true" blood pressure (that is, the average level) than the lower pressures recorded by the patient at home? The fact that the doctor's pressures do predict the degree of risk in hypertensive patients is beyond dispute, but it does not mean that the pressure measured outside the office might not give a better prediction. After all, patients spend much more of their lives at home than in their doctor's office, even the most neurotic ones! But doctors are not known for their modesty, and many don't like to admit the possibility that their readings may be less valid than their patients' readings.

The supremacy of physician readings remained unchallenged until the introduction of a new technique of blood pressure measurement called ambulatory monitoring, which for the first time made it possible to evaluate a patient's pressure over 24 hours, including the whole range of normal daily activities. This revolutionary technique, although first developed in the 1960s, did not find any widespread application for about 20 years, and is only now beginning to be accepted as a clinically useful tool. Most insurance companies do not reimburse patients for its cost (anywhere between $150 and $300), which has restricted its use.

When we started to use these monitors in our research program we undertook a study of 100 patients, whom we trained to monitor their blood pressure at home, and who also wore an ambulatory monitor for 24 hours, to see whether the patients' readings, made at home, or the doctors', made in the office, were closer to the average 24-hour levels recorded by the ambulatory monitor. Somewhat to our consternation, we found that indeed the patients' recordings were closer to the 24-hour levels than the doctors', which tended to be the highest of the three sets of measurements.

In another study of 291 patients, we made another set of comparisons, this time using readings taken by a technician, as well as by a doctor. The technician's readings were closer to the 24-hour level than the doctors', which again were higher than the other two measurements. In this case the physical setting was the same, and the only tenable explanation for the differences in the readings was that the people taking them had different psychological effects on the patients.

I could quote numerous other studies that have obtained similar findings, but the bottom line is that blood pressure readings taken by doctors tend to significantly overestimate a patient's true blood pressure. If this overestimation was the same for everyone, it wouldn't matter very much, because the doctor's readings would still provide an accurate estimate of the level of blood pressure at other times, but unfortunately this is not the case. Although in most patients the doctor's readings are higher than the true blood pressure, in others they are the same, and in a few they are actually lower. The latter case, which is the opposite of white-coat hypertension, is a small but interesting group, some of whom are smokers. Smoking raises blood pressure, but most patients don't smoke in their doctor's office. This explains why the doctor's readings (taken while they're not smoking) may be lower than the ambulatory readings (taken while they are smoking).

WHAT IS WHITE-COAT HYPERTENSION?

When we became aware of the discrepancy between clinic and ambulatory blood pressures, we thought it worthwhile to ask the question: How many patients who are judged to be hypertensive on the basis of their clinic blood pressures in fact have normal blood pressures at other times? To answer this, we needed to know what a normal 24-hour blood pressure is. Like any other definition of normotension and hypertension, this is arbitrary, but we chose a level of 134/90 mm Hg based on a study of ambulatory blood pressure in normal individuals. We found that about 20 percent of our patients with mild hypertension (diastolic pressures in the clinic between 90 and 104 mm Hg) had ambulatory pressures which were unequivocally normal. These were the people we designated as having white-coat hypertension.

An important question about white-coat hypertension is whether the rise of blood pressure that occurs during an office visit is merely a reflection of the response to stress in general. Obviously, its implications could be very different if the same increase of blood pressure occurred during the stresses of daily life, as opposed to being an idiosyncratic response to your doctor. We examined this question in our study, and did not find any evidence that our patients with white-coat hypertension were more likely to show an exaggerated blood pressure response at work. Other researchers have studied this question in a different way, by examining the blood pressure response of patients with white-coat hypertension to standardized stressful situations in the laboratory. One such situation that is commonly used is called the cold pressor test. You put one hand into ice water for one minute, which is quite painful and produces a marked increase in blood pressure. Another challenge is to perform mental arithmetic—for example, by verbally subtracting 13's from a large number. In neither of these cases do patients with white-coat hypertension show any consistently bigger response than other people. In other words, it seems that the white-coat phenomenon is indeed largely confined to the doctor's office.

HOW COMMON IS WHITE-COAT HYPERTENSION?

There are by now several published studies of white-coat hypertension, and the consensus is that it is quite common, occurring in about 20 percent of hypertensive patients. Actually, the increase in blood pressure in a doctor's office occurs no less frequently in patients with sustained hypertension, but the implications are different, because these people are still hypertensive outside the doctor's office.

White-coat hypertension can occur in just about anyone. We find it to be a little commoner in women than in men, and it's surprisingly common in older people. In one study 40 percent of hypertensives over the age of 65 had white-coat hypertension.

How Do I Know If I Have White-Coat Hypertension?

Like any other form of hypertension, white-coat hypertension can be diagnosed only by measuring the blood pressure. There is no evidence that people who have it are generally any more anxious or neurotic than other people, except perhaps when seeing their doctor. Some of my patients have successful and demanding careers, and do not necessarily show any manifestations of anxiety when I take their blood pressure.

At the very least, diagnosing white-coat hypertension involves a series of office visits together with some measurements made outside the office. It should be emphasized that one office visit is not enough, because in many people the blood pressure measured on subsequent visits will be lower than on the first occasion. If the blood pressure measured at home appears to be normal, the next step would be to wear an ambulatory monitor for 24 hours to check whether the pressure is still normal at work.

The Causes of White-Coat Hypertension

The simplest explanation for the phenomenon of white-coat hypertension is that it occurs because people get anxious when they see their doctor, and this makes the blood pressure go up. While this certainly can explain why the blood pressure is higher at the initial visit than on later ones, why should this increase of pressure go on happening year after year in some people? I have one patient whom I have been seeing regularly for the past ten years, who measures her pressure at home, and in whom I still get readings that are as much as 50 mm Hg higher than she gets at home. She knows by now that I am not going to recommend any change in her treatment simply on the basis of the readings that I get, so why does her pressure continue to go up every time she sees me?

We think that the basis for white-coat hypertension lies in the doctor-patient relationship, and the fact that the doctor is perceived as a potentially threatening figure who is the harbinger of bad news for the patient. There have been some interesting studies performed in the past that support the idea that being exposed to an authoritarian figure can indeed make your blood pressure increase. One example is a study of army recruits performed 25 years ago, in which the blood pressure response to a series of challenges was measured. The experiment was conducted by either a captain or a private. Although the procedure was exactly the same in the two cases, the blood pressure responses were significantly greater when the experimenter was the captain. A series of studies along similar lines has been carried out by Dr. James Lynch, who investigated the effects of talking on blood pressure. The mere process of talking makes the pressure increase, but of greater interest is the effect of who you're talking to: if it's someone you regard as being of high status, your pressure is likely to increase more than if it's someone of lower status.

One way in which we envision white-coat hypertension developing goes like this. When you first see a doctor, even if it's for a routine examination, you are naturally anxious that he or she will find something wrong, so your blood pressure is likely to be a bit higher than at other times. Your doctor measures your pressure, and then looks concerned, and tells you that your pressure is high and that this means you may be at increased risk of having a stroke or a heart attack. So you need to make another appointment to come and have it checked again, to see if it's consistently high. You do this, and when you come back you're even more anxious, with the result that your pressure is now higher, not lower. With repeated visits, the pattern becomes more ingrained.

That this actually occurs has been very nicely demonstrated in a study performed by Dr. Morten Rostrup in Norway. He measured the blood pressure of a number of army recruits aged in their twenties, and identified those who had high readings. These he divided into two groups, one of which was sent a letter telling them that their blood pressure was high and needed to be rechecked, while the others were simply told that their blood pressure needed to be measured again. When the two groups showed up two weeks later for their second visit, the pressure of the first group was 15 mm Hg higher than the pressure of the second group. This difference persisted throughout a 45-minute period of testing, and the blood pressure of the first group also showed a bigger increase during mental challenge. These dramatic differences in pressure could be explained only by what the two groups had been told in the letters.

We developed the idea that white-coat hypertension may be a manifestation of what is known scientifically as *classical* or *Pavlovian conditioning,* after the Russian physiologist Ivan Pavlov. When a dog is shown a piece of meat, it starts to salivate. One of Pavlov's experiments was to show the dog a red oval just before it was shown the food, so that the dog learned to associate the oval with the appearance of food. After a few trials the dog would begin to salivate even when the oval was shown without any food. Pavlov called this process "conditioning."

The same process almost certainly happens in people, although it has been given surprisingly little credence by the medical profession. One relatively well-established example, which is of relevance to the phenomenon of white-coat hypertension, occurs in patients with cancer who are treated with a series of intravenous injections of anticancer drugs (referred to as adjuvant therapy), which have the distressing side effect of inducing nausea and vomiting. After a few such injections some patients actually vomit before they receive the injection. In this case the patient learns to associate the appearance of the doctor with the subsequent nausea and vomiting. The phenomenon was vividly described by Dr. Ajit Divgi in a letter he wrote to the *New England Journal of Medicine:*

> I am an oncologist in clinical practice in Milwaukee, and I saw a patient at a local shopping mall three years after she had received adjuvant therapy for breast cancer. She promptly threw up after seeing me, and I can assure you I am not that bad to look at. I presume that this happened because of a conditioned reflex associated with her past chemotherapy.

The equivalent situation with white-coat hypertension would be as follows: the stimulus that is originally responsible for the increase of blood pressure is the fear associated with seeing the doctor for the first time, and after a few visits the pressure may continue to go up even in the absence of any overt fear.

DOES WHITE-COAT HYPERTENSION AFFECT THE RISK OF HEART DISEASE AND STROKE?

This, of course, is the big question, and one to which unfortunately we don't yet have a definitive answer. What we need to do is to follow the progress of patients with white-coat hypertension to see if they are indeed less likely to have strokes and heart attacks than people with sustained hypertension. Such evidence as is available, however, suggests that the risk is low. Several studies have looked to see whether the damage inflicted by hypertension is less in patients with white-coat hypertension than in those whose blood pressure remains persistently high and have generally found it to be less. Thus, the hearts of patients with white-coat hypertension do not show the same degree of enlargement as in patients with sustained hypertension, and no signs of brain damage show up on magnetic resonance imaging (MRI) scans.

Our own data, and those of other researchers, also indicate that the risk of stroke and heart attack is probably relatively low in patients with white-coat hypertension, although these findings are still preliminary, and not yet accepted as gospel by most doctors. The most conclusive evidence has come from an Italian study conducted by Dr. Paolo Verdecchia, who followed the course of more than a thousand hypertensive patients for three years and found that the risk of heart disease was the same in the ones with white-coat hypertension as in people with normal blood pressure, and much lower than in the ones whose blood pressure remained high all the time. I should also emphasize that having a diagnosis of white-coat hypertension does not confer immortality; patients with white-coat hypertension can have strokes and heart attacks just like anybody else if they smoke and have a high cholesterol.

SHOULD I TAKE MEDICATION IF I HAVE WHITE-COAT HYPERTENSION?

Doctors are currently divided on this issue. The politically correct policy is that treatment should be based on the doctor's readings, on the assumption that only doctors know how to measure blood pressure properly. My own view is that if your blood pressure can be shown to be persistently normal outside the doctor's office (for example, below 135 to 140 systolic, and 85 to 90 diastolic), and if you have no evidence of damage from high blood pressure (for example, enlargement of your heart), taking drugs to control your pressure may not be necessary.

Indeed, our own studies and those of others have shown that if your doctor does follow the traditional guidelines and prescribe treatment, one of two things may happen. First, the drug may lower the pressure only in the clinic, and have no effect at other times (what we would regard as a placebo effect), or second, it might lower the pressure persistently, in which case the blood pressure might be too low most of the time, and cause side effects such as dizziness and weakness.

SUMMARY

• Your blood pressure is likely to be higher in your doctor's office than when you're at home.

• White-coat hypertension means that your blood pressure is high only when you are in the doctor's office, and is normal when you're at home or at work.

• It is quite common, and occurs in about 20 percent of hypertensive people.

• People who have it are not generally more anxious or neurotic than others.

• It can only be diagnosed by taking a series of blood pressure measurements away from your doctor's office.

• Although not all doctors agree, you probably do not need to take blood-pressure-lowering medication if you have white-coat hypertension.

CHAPTER ELEVEN

HYPERTENSION AND HEART DISEASE IN WOMEN

The subject of women and heart disease has been much in the news lately. The traditional view is that only men get heart attacks, and many of the studies described in this book have been performed exclusively or predominantly in men.

The myth of women's immunity from heart disease is now being debunked, and it is becoming belatedly recognized that women have been less likely to be given the appropriate treatment (such as coronary artery bypass surgery) than men, even when they complain of the same symptoms. In fact, cardiovascular disease is by far the leading cause of death in women (as in men), and accounts for more than 50 percent of deaths. Nevertheless, it is still true that the death rate is lower in women than in men (at any rate up to the age of 85, by which time most of the men have died).

There are important sex-related differences in the relationships between risk factors and cardiovascular disease, which mean that the treatment strategies should not always be the same for men and for women. In addition, of course, the relevance of menstruation, pregnancy, and the menopause need to be discussed.

ARE DOCTORS BIASED IN THEIR ATTITUDES TOWARD HEART DISEASE IN WOMEN?

The traditional attitude of male doctors toward their female patients complaining of chest pain can be summarized as follows: women are more neurotic than men and complain more; there's no point in doing diagnostic tests because they are less reliable in women; and there's no point in referring them for bypass surgery because they don't do as well as men afterward. While much of this can be dismissed as male chauvinist piggery, there is some justification for all of these statements. Let's look at them in turn. To begin with, in men the first warning of coronary heart disease is typically when they have a heart attack, whereas women are more likely to get angina. Second, it is also true that the diagnostic tests are often less accurate in premenopausal women than in men. The main reason for this is that coronary heart disease is less common in women, so that the chance of getting a false-positive test result (one that looks abnormal but really isn't) is higher. Third, there is also evidence that women get less relief of their symptoms after bypass surgery than men.

There have been a large number of articles in medical journals in the past few years confirming that many doctors do have a biased approach to their female patients. One of the more flagrant examples was a study of thallium exercise stress testing (a relatively accurate test that images the heart with thallium, a radioisotope), in which men were nearly ten times as likely as women to be referred for coronary angiography (the definitive test for coronary heart disease) if the thallium test was abnormal. The women who had symptoms and an abnormal test were more likely to be written off as having psychosomatic pain. Similarly, for those who do go on to have an angiogram, men are nearly four times as likely to be referred for bypass surgery as women.

No self-respecting male doctor would admit to having a prejudiced attitude toward female patients, but these findings demonstrate clearly that it exists, and it has very deep roots. Men are supposed to be macho and stoic, so when they complain of pain, it's assumed to be real.

As a woman, you should be aware of this situation, if you're not already. You're entitled to be taken seriously, and if you think your doctor is being patronizing or offhand with you, find another. It will probably have to be another man, because although about 50 percent of medical students are women, only 20 percent of practicing physicians are, and few of them go into cardiology.

BLOOD PRESSURE CHANGES WITH AGE IN WOMEN

For most of their lives, women have a slightly lower average blood pressure than men, but in both sexes there is a gradual increase with age. At about 50, corresponding to the age of the menopause, women catch up with men, and at older ages tend to have somewhat higher pressures. There is some dispute as to whether there is an accelerated increase associated with the menopause, or whether it merely represents the gradual increase with aging. Most of the evidence would favor the latter view.

BLOOD PRESSURE AS A RISK FACTOR FOR CARDIOVASCULAR DISEASE IN WOMEN

Although blood pressure is a risk factor for heart disease and stroke in both sexes, at any level of blood pressure the risk of coronary heart disease is lower in women than in men, at any rate up to the age of the menopause.

SHOULD HIGH BLOOD PRESSURE BE TREATED DIFFERENTLY IN WOMEN THAN IN MEN?

Most of the early trials of the benefits of treating hypertension were carried out in men. The first one to address the issue of whether these benefits were the same for women was the Hypertension Detection and Follow-up Program (HDFP), which was a randomized trial involving 10,940 subjects, of whom 46 percent were women and 44 percent black. Overall, the results of this trial were very positive: mortality was reduced by about 20 percent. One of the most surprising findings, which was glossed over by the organizers of the trial, was that while in black women the mortality was reduced by a hefty 28 percent as a result of treatment, in white women it was 2 percent *higher* than in the control group. Another large-scale trial, the Medical Research Council (MRC) Trial, conducted in Britain, included 17,354 subjects, of whom about half were women and almost all were white. Drug treatment lowered mortality by 15 percent in the men, but again appeared to increase it slightly in the women. In the only other trial of the effects of treating mild hypertension in which a comparison of the effects in men and women could be made, the Australian Trial, there appeared to be benefits for both sexes, but the numbers of subjects included in this study were too small to be absolutely sure.

In older patients (above the age of 60), things look a bit more encouraging for women. The European Working Party on High Blood Pressure in the Elderly (EWPHE) trial found that women had an 18 percent reduction in mortality as a result of treatment, whereas in men the reduction was 47 percent.

In a review of these unsettling findings, the Women's Caucus Working Group on Women's Health of the Society of General Internal Medicine came to the following conclusions:

> It is not clear whether white women benefit at all from therapy, or if in fact they are harmed by pharmacological therapy. It is clear, however, that our current practice of treating all hypertensive patients based solely on level of blood pressure without regard to ethnicity or gender is probably based on faulty assumptions and inadequate data.

My own interpretation of these results is that the benefits of treating hypertension are less clear in women than in men because they are at lower risk to begin with, at any rate before the menopause. Therefore women with mild hypertension should not be treated as aggressively as men with the same level of blood pressure. In older patients, where the risks associated with hypertension are more evenly balanced between the sexes, the same criteria for deciding when treatment is appropriate should be used for men and for women.

BLOOD LIPID CHANGES WITH AGE IN WOMEN

Blood LDL cholesterol increases with age in both sexes in much the same way as blood pressure: below the age of 50 women have lower levels, but after 55 their LDL is higher than men's. Women tend to have higher HDLs than men at all ages.

BLOOD LIPIDS IN WOMEN: IS CHOLESTEROL A RISK FACTOR?

The conventional view of cardiovascular risk factors, which is advocated by the American Heart Association and the National Cholesterol Education Program, is that cholesterol is just as important in women as in men, and that they should therefore follow the same dietary recommendations. In fact, this is a myth, and as we'll see, it's HDL, not LDL or total cholesterol, which appears to be more important. The way this misconception came about is not hard to understand: the studies that first established that cholesterol is a risk factor for heart disease were done mostly in men, and since women have lower rates of heart attacks than men anyway, it makes it much harder to show a connection. Furthermore, the studies that showed that lowering cholesterol with drugs also lowered the heart attack rate were also performed in men. I need hardly add that the committees making the recommendations were also predominantly male. So let us look at the facts as they really are.

The most widely quoted study of cardiovascular risk factors, which we've already met several times in this book, is the Framingham Heart Study. When the data for women between the ages of 50 and 80 were analyzed, not only was there no relationship between LDL cholesterol levels and heart attacks, but the women with lower cholesterol had more strokes, and their overall death rate was higher. Another analysis was conducted on the data from the Lipid Research Council study (whose purpose was to investigate the effects of lowering cholesterol). This also showed that in women aged 40 to 69 the total cholesterol did not predict who was at risk of a heart attack.

HDL appears to be a more important risk factor in women than in men. In an Israeli study, women with high HDLs had a low risk of heart disease even when their LDLs and total cholesterol levels were high, a finding that was not apparent in men. A recent analysis, which attracted surprisingly little publicity (perhaps because the result was against currently accepted dogma), examined data from 11 studies involving 120,000 women, and found that there was no consistent relationship between blood total cholesterol and the death rate from cardiovascular disease. Furthermore, women with very low cholesterol (below 160) were at greater risk of dying from noncardiac causes, including cancer.

Triglycerides appear to be more important in women than in men, particularly over the age of 55. And although heart attacks are relatively rare in premenopausal women, when they do occur it is often in women who have a genetically determined combination of high LDL cholesterol, low HDL cholesterol, and high triglycerides.

SHOULD WOMEN RESTRICT THEIR FAT INTAKE?

In women with very high cholesterol, few people would disagree that attempting to reduce the level with diet is appropriate. But in those whose cholesterol is only slightly elevated, the benefits are far from clear. The reason is that the "prudent" low-fat/high-fiber diet that is commonly recommended to lower cholesterol can lower HDL as well as LDL cholesterol. This is illustrated in a study conducted in healthy German women who changed their diet from a regular one in which 40 percent of the total calories came from fat to one with 30 percent from fat. The total cholesterol level fell with the low-fat diet, but so did the HDL, by almost the same amount. Since it appears that HDL is more important in women than LDL, the decrease in HDL could mean that they would be actually worse off by restricting fat. On this basis, there is no good reason to recommend this routinely for the prevention of heart disease in women.

There is another consideration, however. There is a lot of evidence that a low-fat diet may help to protect against some forms of cancer—for example, cancer of the colon and breast. But a recent finding from the Nurses' Health Study reported no association between the intake of fat and fiber and breast cancer in 89,000 women who were followed over an eight-year period.

The bottom line is that while a high-fat intake may not be the villain that it is often thought to be, there is absolutely no evidence that fat has any beneficial effects, and it is unquestionably the most potent source of calories. I would therefore advise moderation, but you don't need to be too obsessed about it unless you're seriously trying to lose weight.

Is Losing Weight as Important in Women as in Men?

As we saw in Chapter 5, body fat tends to be distributed differently in men and in women. Blood HDL cholesterol tends to be lower when the fat is predominantly in the abdomen (as in men) than when it is in the thighs (as in women). And when men lose weight their HDLs go up more, and their LDLs down more than in women.

What this means in practice is that not only is obesity more dangerous from a cardiovascular point of view in men, but also the benefits of losing weight are correspondingly greater.

Should Women Take Medication to Lower Their Cholesterol Levels?

The absence of any relationship between deaths from cardiovascular disease and blood cholesterol levels in women means that, unless your cholesterol is very high (over 300), or you already have heart disease, there is no good reason to try to lower your cholesterol with medication.

THE EFFECTS OF ESTROGENS ON BLOOD PRESSURE AND LIPIDS

The simplest explanation for the differences in blood pressure and the prevalence of heart disease between men and premenopausal women would be the effects of estrogens, hormones that are present in women's blood before the menopause, and whose disappearance is its main cause. Actually, estrogens have relatively little effect on blood pressure, although usually they do tend to lower it a little. They also raise HDL cholesterol.

MENSTRUATION AND BLOOD PRESSURE

Neither blood pressure nor blood lipids shows much change according to the phase of menstruation. You may get symptoms such as weight gain and headache at the time of your period, which you might think mean that your blood pressure is going up, but there's usually no connection.

WHY ARE PREMENOPAUSAL WOMEN PROTECTED AGAINST HEART DISEASE?

Before the menopause cardiovascular disease is about three times commoner in men than in women, but by the age of 70 it's about the same. There are several possible explanations for this difference. Some of the more important ones are listed below.

- Blood pressure is lower in women.
- LDL cholesterol is lower in women.
- HDL cholesterol is higher in women.

ESTROGEN REPLACEMENT THERAPY (ERT) AND CARDIOVASCULAR DISEASE

The need for estrogen replacement therapy after menopause is difficult to assess, because like many other medical decisions, it is a question of balancing the benefits against the risks. Thus, while estrogens are generally thought to reduce the risk of heart disease, they may increase the risk of cancer. Furthermore, in most women they need to be given in conjunction with progestins, which may counteract some of their beneficial effects. ERT has been estimated to reduce the risk of dying from heart disease by 50 percent. It also cuts in half the chances of getting osteoporosis (weakness of the bones), which although rarely fatal is a common and debilitating scourge of postmenopausal women. The downside is that ERT may also double the risk of getting cancer of the uterus, and may cause a slight increase in breast cancer.

Opinions about estrogens fluctuate widely as the results of new studies are published. A recent example is a follow-up of women in the Nurses' Health Study conducted by researchers at Harvard, which found a 30 percent increase in the risk of breast cancer in women who had been taking estrogens for five years or more. This was a much higher rate than previously suspected. The finding was the same whether or not the women were also taking progestins.

In order to evaluate the relative importance of the advantages and disadvantages of ERT we need to know the numbers of women who are likely to be affected by these different diseases. If a disease is very rare, a doubling of the risk of getting it is of little consequence—it's still very rare, and your chances of getting it are very small. If, on the other hand, it's quite common, the same doubling of risk is of much greater consequence.

A careful analysis of the impact of ERT on the actual numbers of women dying from these various diseases has recently been conducted by Dr. Brian Henderson and his colleagues. Their findings are shown in Table 11.1.

Table 11.1. Estimated Effects of ERT on Mortality in Postmenopausal Women

DISEASE	EFFECT ON RISK OF DISEASE	EFFECT ON MORTALITY (DEATHS PER 100,000)
Heart disease	50% decrease	5,250 fewer deaths
Osteoporosis	60% decrease	563 fewer deaths
Cancer of uterus	100% increase	63 more deaths
Cancer of breast	30% increase	561 more deaths

Overall effect = 5,189 fewer deaths

The message is clear: if all women over the age of 50 were to take ERT, there would be 5,189 fewer deaths per 100,000 women. There is a catch, however. Women who die of heart disease tend to be in their seventies and eighties, whereas those who die of cancer tend to be in their fifties and sixties. A recent survey showed that women are much more concerned about developing breast cancer at a relatively young age than about getting heart disease in later life.

The risk of cancer of the uterus occurs because estrogens stimulate the growth of the endometrium (the lining of the uterus), which if unchecked may eventually lead to malignancy. The endometrium is normally sloughed off once a month during menstruation, which reduces this risk. This process can be simulated in postmenopausal women by giving the estrogens cyclically in combination with progestins.

What has been less certain is how the combination of estrogens and progestins affects the risk of the other diseases listed in Table 11.1. According to one recent estimate the combination would yield a partial reduction of the protective effect of estrogens given on their own, such that the overall effect on mortality would result in one third fewer lives being saved than when estrogens are given on their own, but this is really only a guess at this stage.

So far, the only properly controlled study that has investigated the effects of ERT is the National Institutes of Health's Postmenopausal Estrogen/Progestin Interventions (PEPI) Trial, which was conducted in 875 women treated for three years with either placebo (inert treatment) or different combinations of estrogens and progestins. The main finding was that ERT improved the blood lipid profile. LDL (bad) cholesterol was reduced by about 20 percent in all the treatment groups, and HDL (good) cholesterol increased. The best results were obtained with estrogen alone, but the combination with progestins was only slightly less good. There were no increases in blood pressure and no excess cases of cancer as a result of taking ERT.

SHOULD I TAKE ESTROGENS AFTER MENOPAUSE IF I HAVE HIGH BLOOD PRESSURE?

Most doctors do not routinely prescribe ERT for women who have high blood pressure (and I am one of them), but this may change in the near future as more data become available. At this stage I can offer the following advice:

- ERT after menopause is not justifiable on a routine basis at the present time.

- If you are at high risk for heart disease (for example, if you have high blood pressure and high blood lipids), ERT would probably lower your risk.
- The decision to start ERT is best made in liaison with your gynecologist.
- If you've had a hysterectomy, there's no need to take progestins as well as estrogens.
- If you've had breast cancer, or if it runs in your family, you should probably not take ERT.

HIGH BLOOD PRESSURE AND PREGNANCY

High blood pressure is a problem besetting nearly 10 percent of all pregnancies and is important because it can endanger the health of both mother and baby. High blood pressure may appear for the first time in pregnancy (in which case it is called preeclampsia or toxemia), or if already present it may get better.

CHANGES IN BLOOD PRESSURE DURING NORMAL PREGNANCY

During a normal pregnancy the diastolic blood pressure goes down by about 5 to 10 mm Hg, reaching its lowest point in the middle of the pregnancy, and gradually increasing to approximately the nonpregnant level just before the baby is born. Systolic pressure doesn't change much. The reason for this change is that the blood vessels in the uterus open up in order to supply nutrients to the placenta and the developing fetus. This dilation would lower the pressure even more if it were not for the fact that the heart pumps more blood during pregnancy.

PREECLAMPSIA (TOXEMIA OF PREGNANCY)

In some women the blood pressure may increase during the later stages of pregnancy (20 weeks or more), sometimes in association with swelling of the ankles. There's also a marked gain in weight, which is not due to overeating, but to retention of salt and water. This condition has various names, the commonest being preeclampsia. The reason for this name is that if untreated it may proceed to the more severe condition of eclampsia, characterized by very high blood pressure, headaches, and convulsions. It's also known as hypertension of pregnancy or toxemia (which literally means blood poisoning). Having blood pressure measured regularly during pregnancy is, hence, very important for all women, as is testing the urine for protein (protein in the urine being another manifestation). The specific criteria used to diagnose preeclampsia are as follows:

- An increase in systolic pressure of 30 mm Hg
- An increase in diastolic pressure of 15 mm Hg
- A blood pressure of 140/90 mm Hg

We don't know what causes preeclampsia, but it may be related to a failure of the uterus to develop normally during pregnancy. It's most likely to occur during first pregnancies, and does not necessarily recur with subsequent ones. Other risk factors for its occurrence include diabetes, previous high blood pressure, and a twin pregnancy. And as mysteriously as it develops during pregnancy, equally mysteriously it goes away after delivery.

It's very important that proper treatment be given, which can greatly reduce the risks of harm to both the mother and the baby. This consists of bed rest (often in hospital), medications, and, if necessary, early delivery of the baby.

IS IT SAFE TO GET PREGNANT IF I ALREADY HAVE HIGH BLOOD PRESSURE?

Most women with mild or moderate hypertension can go through pregnancy with little problem, although it may require a change of medications, because there are some (such as angiotensin converting enzyme inhibitors) that are known to cause fetal damage.

If you have kidney disease as well, you should seek out a physician who is experienced in the management of high blood pressure during pregnancy, because here the risks may be higher.

HOW HIGH BLOOD PRESSURE DURING PREGNANCY IS MANAGED

Because of the potentially harmful effects of medications on the developing fetus, the emphasis in the management of high blood pressure during pregnancy is on nondrug treatment. The general principles are as follows:

- *Restriction of Activity.* Bed rest is one way of lowering blood pressure that has traditionally been used for treating hypertension of pregnancy, and blood flow to the uterus is higher when you are lying down than when standing. In mild cases, this simply means getting off your feet for a few hours each day, but in severe cases it may require admission to hospital. In the majority of cases, this will result in a lower blood pressure and in an improvement of the ankle swelling.
- *Diet.* Salt restriction is usually not recommended during pregnancy, because hypertension in pregnancy is caused by excessive constriction of the arteries, and restriction of salt would further impair the flow of blood to the uterus. However, if you're already on a low-salt diet before you become pregnant, this doesn't mean that you should eat more salt. It may be a good idea to increase your calcium intake, since preeclampsia seems to be commoner in women who eat little calcium.
- *Smoking and Drinking.* Both of these are strongly discouraged, because they can damage the baby irreversibly (for example, via fetal alcohol syndrome). Alcohol can also raise blood pressure in the mother.
- *Home Blood Pressure Monitoring.* This procedure is described in detail in Chapter 17. Although most obstetricians do not recommend using it, if your blood pressure is of concern while you're pregnant, it can be very useful, and help your doctor to decide if you're getting enough rest, for example.

DRUG TREATMENT OF HYPERTENSION DURING PREGNANCY

If the measures described above are not successful in controlling the blood pressure, you will need to start taking antihypertensive medication. And if you're already taking it before you became pregnant, you're likely to need to continue it. The objectives of this treatment are twofold: to keep the mother's blood pressure down and to optimize the growth of the baby. Drugs taken by the mother usually get into the baby's circulation, and everyone remembers the damage done by thalidomide, a tranquilizer widely prescribed to pregnant women in Europe, which resulted in the birth of limbless babies. Of the antihypertensive drugs, only captopril has been shown to cause major problems.

Fortunately, there are some antihypertensive drugs that we know are quite safe for pregnant women to take. Let's look at what is known about the safety of the different types of antihypertensive medications. If you want to know more about how these drugs work, refer to Chapter 22.

Methyldopa. This agent, which has been available for many years, is distinctly unfashionable for treating most people with hypertension, but for pregnant women it is tried and true. It is, in fact, the only medication that has been definitely proved to better the outlook for both mother and child. This was the finding of a study conducted by Dr. Christopher Redman in England, and published in 1976.

Diuretics. Although they are widely and routinely used for treating most types of hypertension, diuretics are not usually favored for treating hypertension of pregnancy, for the same reason that we don't recommend salt restriction. However, this reason is more theoretical than factual, and diuretics may be needed to control the excessive ankle swelling that sometimes accompanies preeclampsia.

Beta Blockers. There is now sufficient experience with these agents to say that as a group they are safe, although there has been some suspicion that they may slow fetal growth.

Calcium-Channel Blockers. Not a lot is known about their long-term safety when used in pregnant women, although they have been widely used, particularly in Europe. The most experience has been with nifedipine (Procardia).

Vasodilators (Hydralazine). Like methyldopa, hydralazine is one of the oldest antihypertensive agents, which is little used except during pregnancy. Here its main use is as a temporary measure for bringing down the blood pressure in an emergency, usually in a hospital setting.

Angiotensin Converting Enzyme (ACE) Inhibitors. This is one group of agents that should never be used in pregnant women, because they can cause severe damage to the baby.

SHOULD I TRY TO LOSE WEIGHT DURING PREGNANCY?

If you're obese, hypertensive, and pregnant, this is not the time to start that weight-reducing diet. It's very important to eat a well-balanced diet while you're pregnant, so that your baby is not affected by any nutritional deficiencies. Your obstetrician will tell you how much weight you should gain during pregnancy.

CAN I CONTINUE TO EXERCISE?

Regular aerobic exercise is in general beneficial for people with high blood pressure, and this probably also applies during the early stages of pregnancy. If you develop preeclampsia during the later stages, however, your doctor may ask you to restrict your physical activity.

SHOULD I TAKE ASPIRIN?

Aspirin is probably the most commonly used medicine during pregnancy. Opinions on its risks and benefits have veered widely over the past few years, and the final word is not yet in. Earlier in this century aspirin was advocated for the relief of all pregnancy-related symptoms, but later on there were concerns that regular use of it might prolong pregnancy and result in babies of low birth weight. About twenty years ago it was suggested that aspirin might help to prevent preeclampsia, or hypertension associated with pregnancy, and since that time several small studies have lent support to this idea. However, the largest and most recent study, which was conducted in Italy, did not find any benefit when aspirin was given to women who were thought to be at high risk of developing hypertension during pregnancy.

At the present time, therefore, there is no reason to recommend taking aspirin routinely. If, however, your doctor considers you to be at high risk of developing preeclampsia, he or she may recommend that you take it.

IS IT SAFE TO BREAST-FEED WHILE TAKING MEDICATION?

If you were taking antihypertensive medications before you were pregnant, you're almost certain to need to continue them afterward. The snag here is that the medication will find its way into your breast milk, and it's not clear what effect this will have on your baby's blood pressure or further development. It may be possible to withhold the medication for a few months if your hypertension is mild, but if it's not, and particularly if you take more than one kind of medication, breast-feeding is not a good idea.

SUMMARY

• Heart disease is the biggest cause of death in women, just as in men.

• Women have lower blood pressure and less heart disease than men until menopause, after which they catch up.

• Because they are at lower risk than men to begin with, premenopausal women need not have their blood pressure treated as aggressively as men.

• Total and LDL cholesterol are less important as risk factors in women than in men, while HDL cholesterol and triglycerides are more important in women.

• Estrogens may be one reason why premenopausal women enjoy protection from cardiovascular disease; administration of estrogens after menopause may help to continue this protection, but with a small increased risk of breast cancer.

• Unless you have had a hysterectomy, estrogen replacement therapy needs to be combined with progestins to prevent cancer of the uterus. Progestins may counteract some of the beneficial effects of estrogens.

• I do not at present recommend estrogen replacement therapy routinely for all hypertensive women after menopause.

• High blood pressure can begin during pregnancy, and puts both mother and baby at risk. It can be treated, however, if necessary, with medications.

CHAPTER TWELVE

HIGH BLOOD PRESSURE IN THE ELDERLY

Until very recently, we really didn't know what to do about high blood pressure in old people, who in this context are defined as anyone over the age of 65. This was because, although we did know that hypertension is a risk factor for strokes and heart attacks in older people just as in younger ones, it was not known whether treating the blood pressure would lower this risk. In the past five years there have been several large-scale clinical trials of treatment of hypertension in the elderly that have shown very conclusively that treatment is beneficial, if anything more so than in younger patients. I will describe these in this chapter, and also some of the ways in which hypertension in the elderly differs from hypertension in people below the age of 65, with particular reference to what is called systolic hypertension of the elderly.

HOW AGING AFFECTS BLOOD PRESSURE

It used to be said that a normal blood pressure is 100 plus your age. While it is certainly true that blood pressure does tend to increase as we grow older, it does not necessarily follow that this is "normal," if by "normal" you mean healthy. And in fact the rise of blood pressure with age is by no means inevitable or universal. It doesn't occur in many so-called primitive societies, although it must be admitted that their life expectancy is often not as long as ours, because they die from infections and malnutrition. And in a study of nuns living in a secluded convent in Italy it was found that the nuns' blood pressures showed less increase with age than the blood pressures of women living in the world outside.

So perhaps the stresses and strains of daily life in modern society contribute to the increase of blood pressure with age.

SYSTOLIC HYPERTENSION OF THE ELDERLY

Most people with high blood pressure have elevations of both systolic and diastolic pressure, but in some older people the systolic pressure may be high (above 160 mm Hg) while the diastolic is quite normal (below 90). This is referred to as isolated systolic hypertension, and affects about 20 percent of people over the age of 70. It used to be thought that the diastolic pressure is more important than the systolic, but this is wrong, and in fact the systolic pressure is somewhat more important in predicting your risk.

The mechanism underlying systolic hypertension is different from the mechanism of the hypertension that occurs in younger people. As we grow older, our arteries grow stiffer and lose their elasticity. When the heart pumps blood into the aorta (the large artery leaving the heart) of a young person, it expands to accommodate the extra volume of blood, which means that the pressure goes up by only a moderate amount. But an older and stiffer aorta cannot expand as much, so that there is a greater surge of pressure. This peak of pressure is, of course, the systolic pressure.

WHAT ARE THE BENEFITS OF TREATING HYPERTENSION IN THE ELDERLY?

The original trials of the effects of treating hypertension were almost all conducted in patients below the age of 65, so that despite the fact that we knew that older people were at increased risk from their blood pressure, we couldn't be sure that treating it would lower the risk. In the past few years there have been several large-scale trials, mostly conducted in Europe, which have laid these doubts to rest. One of the most widely publicized was the SHEP (Systolic Hypertension of the Elderly Program) study, which was carried out in the United States. More than 4,000 patients were entered into the trial. To be eligible, they had to be at least 65 years old and to have a systolic pressure greater than 160 and a diastolic pressure less than 90 mm Hg. Patients were then randomly allocated to one of two groups: those in the treatment group were prescribed a daily diuretic pill, while those in the control group were given a placebo (inert pill). At the end of five years there were striking results—strokes were decreased by 36 percent in the treated group, and heart attacks by 27 percent. One of the interesting things about SHEP and some of the other trials conducted in the elderly was that drug treatment was almost as effective in preventing heart attacks as strokes; in trials conducted in younger patients strokes were cut by 50 percent, but heart attacks by only 10 percent.

IS THE TREATMENT THE SAME AS IN YOUNGER PATIENTS?

When treatment of high blood pressure in older patients is prescribed, it's usually medication rather than exercise or a change of diet, although there's no evidence that these would be any less effective in the elderly. There has actually been very little investigation of nondrug forms of treatment. The same drugs are used as in younger patients. Diuretics are usually chosen first, because they were the drugs used in most of the treatment trials such as SHEP. I tend to prescribe beta blockers less in older patients.

HIGH BLOOD PRESSURE IN THE VERY OLD

The studies that have shown the benefits of lowering the blood pressure of elderly patients have been restricted to people below the age of 85. After that, all bets are off. In fact, several studies have shown that in the very old, high blood pressure may not be such a bad thing. One, which was conducted in the city of Tampere in Finland in people aged from 84 to 88 years, found that the lowest mortality occurred in those whose systolic pressure was between 140 and 170 mm Hg, and diastolic between 70 and 100 mm Hg. When the pressure was either below or above these levels, the death rate from cardiovascular disease was higher. Other studies have found generally similar results.

The lesson here is that if you make it to the age of 85, you're a survivor, and you've already exceeded the average life expectancy. Any attempts by doctors to prolong it further by lowering your blood pressure are likely to prove fruitless. If you're already taking medication, however, and it's not causing any problems, I would not recommend stopping it.

HIGH BLOOD CHOLESTEROL IN THE ELDERLY—THE BULLET MISSED

The National Cholesterol Education Program recommends that "high-risk elderly patients who are otherwise in good health are candidates for cholesterol-lowering therapy." If their recommendations were followed, huge numbers of healthy older people (38 percent of men and 48 percent of women) between the ages of 65 and 74 would be prescribed expensive medication that they do not need, and that might also be positively harmful.

The reason I say that the NCEP recommendations are wrong is that when you examine the data on cholesterol and heart disease in the old it is clear that cholesterol becomes of progressively less importance as a risk factor after the age of 60. This was highlighted by a recent study (published in the *Journal of the American Medical Association*) conducted on 1,000 healthy residents of New Haven, Connecticut, aged 70 or more, all of whom had their cholesterol measured at the start of the study. Over the next four years there was absolutely no connection between the total or HDL cholesterol levels and the chance of dying or having a heart attack.

In an editorial accompanying this report two respected epidemiologists (Stephen Hulley and Thomas Newman) suggested that healthy people over the age of 70 do not need to have their cholesterol checked, let alone treated. For those between 65 and 70 screening and treatment are appropriate in people who are at high risk of heart disease. I agree with these recommendations. What they mean in practice is that if you are over 65 and have a high cholesterol (and perhaps also high blood pressure), but are otherwise healthy, it's not worth taking cholesterol-lowering medication. If, however, you've already had heart problems or a stroke, taking the medication may help to keep you out of further trouble.

The potential downside to taking the medication if you don't really need it is that it could be harmful. Several epidemiological studies have shown that older people with low cholesterol tend to have a higher death rate from noncardiovascular causes than people with higher cholesterol (see Chapter 2 for more about this), so that it is possible that taking the medication may reduce your risk of heart disease, while increasing it for other types of disease. If your risk of heart disease is very high, the benefits of taking medication may outweigh the risks, but if it's not, they may balance out. Like many other subjects discussed in this book, it's a trade-off.

SUMMARY

• Systolic blood pressure increases with age more than diastolic, because our arteries gradually lose their elasticity.

• Systolic hypertension of the elderly increases the risk of cardio-vascular disease, but lowering the blood pressure with medication can reduce this risk.

• Above the age of 85, high blood pressure appears to be no longer a risk factor, so there's no justification to start treating it.

CHAPTER THIRTEEN

RACE AND HIGH BLOOD PRESSURE

One of the major unresolved issues in hypertension is the striking effect of race: high blood pressure is approximately twice as common in blacks as in whites. The big question is whether this is due to genetic or environmental reasons. There have been many suggestions that the physiological processes regulating blood pressure are different in blacks and whites, and that the effectiveness of different types of blood-pressure-lowering medications may not be the same. Blacks in the United States tend to be subjected to more stress than whites, and this may also be a factor. There are also unexplained racial differences in the consequences of hypertension. We'll discuss all of these issues in this chapter.

WHY IS HYPERTENSION MORE COMMON IN BLACKS THAN WHITES?

Although blacks in the United States have consistently higher blood pressure than whites, this pattern is not the same in all other parts of the world. In Africa, blood pressure tends to be relatively low in rural areas and high in the cities. And a study of factory workers in Birmingham, England, found no difference in the pressures of black and white workers. A group that is at particular risk of developing high blood pressure (in England just as much as in the United States) is black women, in whom obesity plays a major role. Since these populations share a common African origin and the same genetic background, it is unlikely that heredity can account for all of the racial differences seen in the United States. Nonetheless, heredity is an important cause of high blood pressure in blacks just as in whites, so if you're black and both your parents have high blood pressure, you have an increased chance of getting it yourself.

One possible explanation might be that blacks use more salt than whites. This has not been found to be the case, although blacks do tend to ingest less potassium, and according to some studies, less calcium. Both of these would tend to be associated with higher blood pressure.

There seems to be something about the modern Western lifestyle that raises blood pressure in blacks just as much as in whites. One study noted that when a group of Kenyan tribesmen migrated from their rural village to the city of Nairobi, their blood pressures increased markedly. One of the most important studies of the effects of the urban environment on blood pressure was conducted by Dr. Ernest Harburg and his colleagues in Detroit, who found the highest blood pressures in black males living in "high-stress" neighborhoods, which were characterized by low income, high unemployment, and high crime rates. Another factor that was found to be associated with higher pressures was suppressed anger. Harburg also found that men with darker skin had higher pressures than those with pale skin. The skin color of American blacks is determined genetically, and reflects how much their ancestry is African rather than European. However, it is also possible that blacks with darker skin are subjected to more stress in the form of racial discrimination than those with pale skin. This question has to some extent been resolved by a recent study performed in three U.S. cities—Savannah, Georgia; Hagerstown, Maryland; and Pueblo, Colorado—which confirmed the association between high blood pressure and dark skin, but only in people of lower socioeconomic status. The simplest explanation of this finding is that people at the lower end of the social scale are less able to cope with the stress associated with darker skin color. If the association between blood pressure and skin color was genetic, it should have been evident in all social classes. Thus some of the high blood pressure in blacks can be attributed to stress.

Secondary or curable forms of hypertension (described in Chapter 14) are less common in blacks than in whites.

RACIAL DIFFERENCES IN THE PROCESSES REGULATING BLOOD PRESSURE

A great deal of effort has gone into attempts to identify differences in the physiological processes controlling blood pressure. One that has emerged with some consistency is salt sensitivity: there is a much greater chance that your blood pressure will respond to a change in salt intake if you're black than if you're white. Low-renin hypertension is relatively common in blacks. This is a type of hypertension that is thought to be caused by salt retention, and blacks tend to be more salt-sensitive than whites (see Chapter 3 for a description of this).

RACIAL DIFFERENCES IN THE CONSEQUENCES OF HYPERTENSION

Whatever your skin color, the major consequences of untreated hypertension are stroke, heart attack, and kidney disease. Overall, blacks have more cardiovascular disease than whites, but this is because they have more hypertension. For the same level of blood pressure, blacks are no worse off than whites. The relative frequency of the complications resulting from high blood pressure is not the same, however. Strokes are at least as common in blacks as in whites, but heart attacks are commoner in whites. This may be because blood cholesterol and triglyceride levels are lower in blacks, and high-density lipoprotein levels higher, and these factors offset the effects of the high blood pressure. Nevertheless, coronary heart disease is the leading cause of death in blacks just as it is in whites.

The kidneys seem to be especially vulnerable to the effects of hypertension in black individuals, and kidney failure, which can ultimately lead to the need for dialysis, is commoner than in whites. Even in people with normal blood pressure, the decline of kidney function that is associated with increased age is more marked in blacks than in whites.

SHOULD HYPERTENSION BE TREATED DIFFERENTLY IN BLACKS AND WHITES?

The two principal forms of nondrug treatment, weight reduction and salt restriction, are at least as important in blacks as in whites. Blacks tend to be a little more salt-sensitive than whites (see Chapter 3 for a description of this).

There are some minor differences in the responses to antihypertensive drug treatment: the two most widely used classes of agents are beta blockers and diuretics, and blacks tend to show a slightly better response to the latter, while whites do better with the former. The other class of drug where there also seems to be a racial difference is the an-giotensin converting enzyme inhibitors (ACE inhibitors), where again whites tend to show a bigger response than blacks.

These differences can all be attributed to the fact that low-renin hypertension is commoner in blacks, and high-renin hypertension in whites. Beta blockers and ACE inhibitors work by blocking the effects of renin on blood pressure, so they are most effective when the level of renin is high. Conversely, diuretics work best when there is salt reten-tion and renin is low.

I should emphasize that these are only trends, however. There are many blacks who do well with both beta blockers and ACE inhibitors, but we wouldn't usually choose these drugs first.

SUMMARY

• High blood pressure is more common in American blacks than in whites: this is probably due to environmental factors rather than to genetics.

• Blacks with hypertension are somewhat less likely to have heart attacks than whites, but more likely to develop kidney problems.

• The treatment of hypertension is basically the same in blacks as in whites, although there are some differences in the responsive-ness to certain medications.

CHAPTER FOURTEEN

SECONDARY OR CURABLE FORMS OF HYPERTENSION

More than 95 percent of patients with high blood pressure have essential hypertension, which means that no specific cause can be found. The other 5 percent are potentially the lucky ones, because many of them have a form of hypertension for which there is the possibility of a permanent cure. It is sometimes referred to as secondary hypertension because the hypertension is secondary to a specific abnormality, usually in the kidneys or adrenal glands; when this abnormality is corrected, the hypertension disappears.

CLUES TO THE PRESENCE OF SECONDARY HYPERTENSION

When your doctor first sees you for a history and physical examination, there are a number of potential clues that may raise the suspicion that you may have one of these rare forms of hypertension. Some of these clues are listed here.

- *Sudden Onset.* Essential hypertension (the common sort) usually develops over several years, and many people give a history of marginally elevated readings before the pressure reaches a level high enough to warrant treating. If, however, you've had annual physical exams, and after having had a pressure of 120/80 mm Hg for many years you are suddenly found to have 180/110, you could have secondary hypertension.
- *Young Age.* Hypertension is rare in children, and when it does occur is usually secondary.

- *Severe Hypertension.* In secondary hypertension the pressure is usually very high.
- *Unusual Symptoms.* Essential hypertension is often detected on a routine physical exam, while people with secondary hypertension often go to their doctor because they have developed severe symptoms such as headache, dizziness, or weakness.
- *Abnormal Finding on Physical Examination.* Blood flowing through a narrowed artery to a kidney may occasionally be audible through a stethoscope placed on the abdomen.

Renovascular Hypertension (Renal Artery Stenosis)

This is by far the commonest type of secondary hypertension, and accounts for about 3 percent of all cases of hypertension. It's caused by a narrowing in one or both renal (kidney) arteries. This reduces the blood pressure and flow in the kidney, which responds by secreting a hormone called renin, which enters the bloodstream and leads to the formation of a second hormone (angiotensin), which causes the blood pressure to go up. This helps to restore the flow to the blocked kidney.

There are two quite distinct causes of renovascular hypertension. The first, which occurs in young people (particularly children and young women), is called fibromuscular dysplasia. There are one or more fibrous constrictions of the artery. An important aspect of this condition is that it hardly ever affects any arteries other than the ones supplying the kidneys. Nobody knows what causes it, although smoking may be a contributory factor; it usually does not run in families.

The second cause is atherosclerosis, sometimes referred to as arteriosclerosis or hardening of the arteries, which is the same process that causes strokes and heart attacks. It occurs in the middle-aged and elderly, and plaques may develop in the renal arteries just as they do in other major vessels. However, when an atheromatous obstruction is detected in a renal artery there is often a chicken-and-egg problem. While a plaque in the renal artery certainly can cause hypertension, hypertension itself can cause or accelerate the development of plaques, so that an atheromatous obstruction in the renal artery cannot always be assumed to be the cause of the hypertension. The important thing to establish is whether the kidney is being starved of blood: if it is, the narrowing is almost certainly contributing to the elevation of the blood pressure.

The way this happens is primarily through the secretion of renin from the affected kidney (see above), and also from the fact that the kidney loses some of its ability to get rid of salt from the body. If only one kidney is involved, the other kidney can handle the extra load, but if both renal arteries are blocked, there will be retention of sodium, which will make the blood pressure go up even more. The affected kidney also begins to shrink, and to lose its capacity to excrete other waste products. Since atheromatous blockages tend to get worse over time, this condition is an important cause of renal failure and the eventual need for dialysis.

Diagnosing Renovascular Hypertension. Even though it's the commonest curable cause of hypertension, most doctors (including myself) do not recommend testing everybody for it. The screening tests are expensive and not wholly reliable, so we usually reserve them for patients in whom there are "clinical clues," as described above. The tests that are used include an abdominal ultrasound test (to examine the size of the kidneys), renal scans (to examine their function), and finally an angiogram. These are all described in more detail in Chapter 16.

Treating Renovascular Hypertension. There are basically three options for treatment of this condition. The first is to keep the blood pressure down with medications. This is generally the least satisfactory, not only because it means continuing to need medications, but also because of the risk of losing a kidney if the narrowing in the artery finally blocks it off completely. The second option is surgery. In the past, this often meant taking out the kidney, but nowadays this is done only as a last resort, when the kidney has already ceased to function (it may still be making renin). The commonest type of operation is a bypass procedure, which involves grafting an artery or vein from another part of the circulation into the renal artery beyond the blockage. Some surgeons actually cut out the plaque that is causing the blockage. The third option is called angioplasty. This procedure first became popular in about 1980, and in many cases is now the preferred treatment. It's done at the same time as an angiogram, and is performed by passing a catheter (a thin plastic tube) with a balloon on its tip through the narrowed portion of the artery. When it's properly positioned the balloon is inflated for 30 seconds, which stretches the narrowing open.

ALDOSTERONE-SECRETING TUMOR (ALDOSTERONOMA)

The clue to this condition is a low blood potassium. Since potassium is part of any routine blood measurement, it should be relatively easy to diagnose, but it's surprising how many patients go for years with low potassium readings before the penny drops. Low potassium is also a side effect of diuretic treatment, so it's often attributed to this.

The culprit is a very small benign tumor of an adrenal gland, which secretes excessive amounts of a hormone called aldosterone, whose function is to regulate the sodium and potassium balance. It acts on the kidney to retain sodium in exchange for potassium, which is excreted in the urine. When aldosterone is produced in excess the retained sodium makes the blood pressure go up, and there is depletion of potassium. Although the blood potassium reading is low, there is no change in the blood sodium concentration, because the extra sodium is diluted by a corresponding retention of water.

Diagnosing Aldosterone-secreting Tumors. The crucial measurement is a combination of a high aldosterone (measured from a urine specimen) and a low renin. Renin indirectly stimulates the secretion of aldosterone, so when renin levels are high (as in renovascular hypertension), aldosterone is also high. However, if the primary disturbance is an excessive secretion of aldosterone, this suppresses the production of renin. The other part of the diagnostic procedure is the visualization of the tumor, which is best performed by a CT (computerized tomography) scan of the adrenal glands.

Treatment. The adrenal gland in which the tumor is growing is removed by a surgical operation, which usually results in a permanent cure of the hypertension.

PHEOCHROMOCYTOMA

This rather indigestible word (pronounced *fee-o-chrome-o-site-o-ma*) describes another type of tumor of the adrenal gland, which secretes another blood-pressure-raising hormone (norepinephrine, and its sister compound epinephrine). This secretion is sometimes intermittent and is manifested by sudden increases in blood pressure, associated with symptoms of sweating and headache. The condition is quite rare, however, and most people with these symptoms do not have a pheochromocytoma.

Diagnosing Pheochromocytoma. There are two steps in the diagnosis: first is the demonstration of increased blood or urine levels of catecholamines (the blanket term for norepinephrine and epinephrine), and second is the visualization of the tumor in one of the adrenal glands, which is done with a CT or MRI (magnetic resonance imaging) scan.

Treatment. Once the tumor has been located, the treatment is by surgical removal of the adrenal gland. This is done only after the effects of the epinephrine and norepinephrine are blocked by appropriate treatment with medications.

SUMMARY

• In less than 5 percent of people with high blood pressure there is a remediable cause, usually some abnormality of the kidneys or adrenal glands.

• These conditions may be suspected if the hypertension comes on very suddenly, at a young age, is of great severity, or is associated with certain symptoms and abnormalities on the routine evaluation.

• The most common type of secondary hypertension is renovascular hypertension, which occurs because of a narrowing in one or both arteries of the kidneys. Relief of the narrowing by surgery or angioplasty may cure or alleviate the hypertension.

• Small tumors of the adrenal gland (called aldosteronomas and pheochromocytomas) raise the blood pressure by secreting hormones into the bloodstream. Both are curable by surgery.

CHAPTER FIFTEEN

LOW BLOOD PRESSURE

Although high blood pressure is much the commoner complaint, there are many people who are convinced that their blood pressure is too low. In general, of course, it's fair to say that the lower your blood pressure the better. One condition where blood pressure is definitely too low, although not all the time, is known as orthostatic or postural hypotension, and is seen mainly in older people, as described later. Many younger people, particularly women (who tend to have lower blood pressure than men), may have systolic pressures in the 90s and diastolics in the 60s. Whether or not this should ever be a cause for concern is the central theme of this chapter.

TRANSIENT LOW BLOOD PRESSURE AND FAINTING

The commonest example of blood pressure being too low, which you may have already experienced, is when you faint. The technical term for this is a *vasovagal episode.* If you lose a lot of blood, or see something very unpleasant, this may trigger a reflex action by the brain, which suddenly slows the heart and dilates the arteries. Your blood pressure falls precipitately, and you fall to the floor. What the purpose of this reflex is has always been something of a mystery; the best explanation I can think of is that if you're losing blood it's better if you're horizontal rather than upright, and fainting is one certain way of getting you there.

When young people faint it's usually nothing to be concerned about, and may simply indicate a very healthy vasovagal reflex. In older people the reflex is usually not so active, so that if fainting does occur, it may have some other less benign cause, such as a change of rhythm of the heart. Another cause may be too much blood-pressure-lowering medication. An example of this might occur when a relatively fast-acting pill is taken at the same time as a meal. In older people the blood pressure may normally fall by several points about an hour after a meal, when blood flow is being diverted to the stomach, and if this is also when the medicine starts to work it could mean trouble. Usually this would not cause an actual blackout, but there could be symptoms of dizziness and lightheadedness. These, of course, are the same symptoms as some people attribute to high blood pressure, and this is one reason why taking your own blood pressure at home (described in Chapter 17) may be so helpful, because it will help your doctor decide whether you're getting too much or too little medication.

CAN CHRONIC LOW BLOOD PRESSURE CAUSE SYMPTOMS?

In Lynn Payer's book *Medicine and Culture,* she describes how the practice of medicine varies in different countries, despite the fact that the countries she chose (the United States, England, Germany, and France) are all advanced westernized societies. One of her more striking examples is the phenomenon of low blood pressure, which in England is referred to as "the German disease." In Germany, people who are found to have low blood pressure all the time (for example 90/50 mm Hg), and who complain of symptoms such as fatigue, are considered to be sick, and are prescribed medication to raise the blood pressure. In the German pharmacopeia there are 85 drugs primarily for the treatment of low blood pressure, virtually none of which would be prescribed by British or American doctors. The German government has statistics on absenteeism from work as a result of low blood pressure. In England, Canada, and the United States low blood pressure is considered to be a sign of excellent health, and those patients who ascribe symptoms to it are written off as being neurotic or crazy. British and American textbooks of medicine simply ignore it, although one Canadian survey found that nearly 10 percent of the population was being treated for it. In Germany it is officially described as "constitutional hypotension," and a typical German textbook describes it more or less as follows:

It exists if the blood pressure is persistently below 110/60 mm Hg in men, or 100/60 mm Hg in women. It is a disturbance of blood pressure control. The leading symptoms are bodily and mental tiredness, giddiness, a tendency to faint, and tightness round the heart. The treatment is systematic bodily exercises and the prescription of vasoconstrictor drugs.

In 1989 an English epidemiologist named John Pemberton wrote a provocative article in the traditionally conservative *British Medical Journal* entitled "Does Constitutional Hypotension Exist?" This was prompted by his having recently visited Germany and being impressed by the different attitudes toward the condition in the two countries. He suggested that perhaps English doctors were ignoring a genuine disorder. Two groups of investigators took up his challenge, and also published their findings in the same journal.

The first was a survey of more than 7,000 adults in England, Scotland, and Wales who had their blood pressures measured, and were asked to fill out a questionnaire describing their symptoms. The results showed that both tiredness and feeling faint were associated with low blood pressure. The authors of the study were careful to point out, however, that these results did not prove that the low blood pressure was the cause of the fatigue, but merely that they often went together. The second study was performed in 10,000 civil servants in London, and came to very similar conclusions. Both dizziness and tiredness were associated with low blood pressure.

So it looks as if the German doctors may be right, and that there is a condition of low blood pressure which is associated with a variety of symptoms. Unfortunately we don't know which is the chicken and which is the egg—does a low blood pressure make you feel tired, or does being tired make your blood pressure go down? It's also quite possible that some unidentified factor is causing both (anemia would be one such example). There seems to be no clear justification from these results to recommend treating the low blood pressure. Since it's certainly true that from the point of view of cardiovascular disease the lower the blood pressure the better, there is a need for a properly controlled study showing that raising the blood pressure with medications actually does make people feel better; so far as I am aware, no such study has been performed.

Postural Hypotension

There is one type of low blood pressure about which there is no debate as to its existence and significance, and that's postural, or orthostatic, hypotension. As its name implies, it is characterized by a fall in blood pressure on standing up, which, if unchecked, may lead to a loss of consciousness. It's not common, and it occurs mainly in older people. It's caused by a deterioration of the blood-pressure-regulating mechanisms.

Normally when we stand up our blood pressure changes very little, because the arteries and veins in our legs constrict, and prevent the blood from pooling in the legs. This happens as a result of a reflex controlled by the brain and the sympathetic nervous system; it's the sympathetic nerves that make the vessels contract. If the sympathetic nerves are not working properly, as is the case in postural hypotension, the blood tends to pool in the legs on standing, and fainting occurs because there's not enough blood left in the system to keep the brain properly perfused. The fainting is different from the vasovagal type seen in young healthy people, because it's very gradual. When people with postural hypotension are horizontal for long periods of time, their blood pressure may go too high.

The treatment of this condition is very difficult. The pooling of blood in the legs can be controlled to some extent by wearing tight-fitting elastic stockings or pantyhose that go up to the waist. These have to be custom-made, and are quite expensive. They are uncomfortable because they are so tight, and they're a nuisance when going to the toilet. The standard medication is Florinef, an analogue of the hormone aldosterone, which makes the kidneys retain sodium and hence keep the blood pressure up. It helps a little, but is no miracle cure. Many other medications have been tried, most of which constrict the blood vessels. None of them work very well, and they all tend to raise the blood pressure even further when the patient is lying flat.

SUMMARY

• Low blood pressure is usually a sign of health rather than of sickness, and although it may be associated with symptoms such as fatigue, it is not necessarily their cause.

• There is no evidence that treating low blood pressure makes people feel any better.

• Postural hypotension is a rare condition that affects mainly older people; the blood pressure goes very low when standing, but is quite high when lying down.

CHAPTER SIXTEEN

THE WORKUP

One of the commonest ways for high blood pressure to be detected is on a routine physical examination, for example, for health insurance. If you are told that you have high blood pressure, you will probably be referred for further evaluation, either by your own doctor or by a specialist. The purpose of this evaluation, or workup, as it's commonly called, is to answer the following questions:

- How high is the pressure?
- What's causing it to go up?
- Has it caused any damage?
- How should it be treated?

Finding the answers to these questions may take a number of visits and several tests, but it's definitely a worthwhile procedure, because high blood pressure is generally a lifelong condition, and you don't want to be prescribed medication unnecessarily, which is not an uncommon event.

WHAT TO EXPECT AT YOUR FIRST VISIT

When you first see your doctor, he or she will conduct a full history and physical examination. You'll probably be asked to describe any symptoms you've had, and how it was first learned that your pressure was up. If you've been feeling perfectly well all along, and have no symptoms to report, don't worry—that's the norm. Your doctor will want to know what level of pressure you've had over the years—when you had previous physical exams, for example, or if you're a woman, how high it was during pregnancy. In most people blood pressure tends to go up gradually with age, but if your pressure has always been normal and suddenly goes to very high levels over a period of six months to a year, it has a very different significance. This may be a clue to an underlying problem with a kidney or adrenal gland.

You'll also be asked about medications you've taken, including both prescribed and over-the-counter medicines. If you've had high blood pressure for some time, and have taken blood-pressure-lowering medications, it's helpful to know whether they did actually lower your pressure (not all medicines work in all patients), and whether you had side effects.

A few prescribed medicines can actually raise blood pressure. The greatest culprit in the past was oral contraceptive medication, but with the lower doses used today this is rarely a problem. Medication taken to abort migraine attacks, such as Cafergot, when taken in very big doses can also raise blood pressure, because it works by constricting blood vessels. Another example is nasal decongestants (see Chapter 25).

Questions about other symptoms and problems will be directed to providing more clues to both the cause and the consequences of the high blood pressure. If, for example, you've experienced episodes of headaches, sweating, and going white in the face, it could be an indication that your hypertension is due to an extremely rare tumor of the adrenal gland (called a pheochromocytoma; see Chapter 14). And if you've begun to get a tight feeling in the chest when you climb a flight of stairs, it may be a sign that the hypertension has affected your heart.

One of the most important determinants of blood pressure is heredity. If one of your parents had high blood pressure, your chance of having it is increased, and if both did, it will be even higher. You'll certainly be asked about your parents' health, therefore. There will also be questions about your lifestyle: if you drink a lot of alcohol, this may raise your blood pressure (see Chapter 7), and if you smoke, this will definitely raise the risk of heart disease (as well as many other diseases). Your diet and exercise habits will also be evaluated (see Chapters 3, 4, and 6).

The physical exam will also focus on the evaluation of the causes and consequences of hypertension. Your doctor will probably take several readings of your blood pressure, from both arms and in different positions: lying, sitting, and standing. I don't pay too much attention to the blood pressure reading at the first visit, however. Many patients are very anxious at this point, which tends to make their blood pressure go up. It often takes several visits to get an idea of what the blood pressure really is.

Routine Lab Tests

The purpose of the lab tests is in general the same as for the history and physical exam—to assess the causes and consequences of the high blood pressure, and also to measure the second of the Big Three risk factors—your blood cholesterol. The basic test is a screening test of blood and urine. Most labs nowadays perform a battery of tests on a blood sample (sometimes called a "chemscreen"), which includes things such as a blood count (which shows whether you're anemic) and tests of liver and kidney function, blood sugar (a measure of diabetes), and electrolytes (most importantly the concentrations of sodium and potassium in the blood). Both of these play an important role in the regulation of blood pressure, and are discussed in more detail in Chapters 3 and 4. Here we will just note that the concentration of sodium in the blood is no indication of whether a person is eating a high- or low-sodium diet. To evaluate that, a 24-hour urine collection is needed (see below). A low blood potassium level may be a clue to a rare cause of hypertension from a small and benign (i.e., not cancerous) tumor of the adrenal gland (see Chapter 14), but much more commonly occurs as a side effect from a class of blood-pressure-lowering medications called diuretics. The cholesterol measurement actually includes three components: cholesterol, HDL, and triglycerides. These are discussed further in Chapter 2. A urine specimen will also be checked, particularly for protein (an indicator of kidney disease) and sugar.

Electrocardiogram

This test is also routine and is the traditional way of seeing if the hypertension has had any effect on the heart. When heart muscle contracts it creates an electrical impulse, which can be detected on the surface of the body. The electrocardiogram (ECG or EKG, for short) is performed by applying six electrodes to the skin on different parts of the chest. Another four are applied to each wrist and ankle. These pick up the electrical signal coming from the heart, which is amplified and recorded on a paper strip. The reason for having so many electrodes is that each one is effectively looking at the heart from a different viewpoint, and the electrical waveform is slightly different in each one. The pattern of waveforms in the different leads provides a lot of information about the structure and function of the heart. For the evaluation of high blood pressure, the two most important things are whether the heart is enlarged, and whether there's any sign of damage from a heart attack. As we'll see shortly, however, the ECG is actually not very accurate for detecting enlargement of the heart.

CHEST X RAY

This is another traditional test, but for the evaluation of high blood pressure is rarely of value. It does show enlargement of the heart, but only when it's very severe.

SOME USEFUL, BUT LESS ROUTINE TESTS

RENIN-SODIUM PROFILE

Although many doctors don't use this test, it actually provides a lot of valuable information, and is easy to do. It involves collecting urine for 24 hours, and then doing a blood test. Renin is a chemical made in the kidney and released into the blood, where it plays a major role in the control of blood pressure (see Chapter 1). Its release is regulated partly by the amount of salt in the body: if you're on a very-low-salt diet your renin is likely to be high, while if you eat pretzels and potato chips all day it will be low. The purpose of the urine collection is to evaluate your salt intake, because most of the salt you eat and drink comes out in the urine. In this way, by measuring the amount of salt (or sodium) in the urine, it is possible to see if your renin level is appropriate for your salt intake. This is why the test is known as the renin-sodium profile. Some people make a lot of renin even when they're not on a low-salt diet, in which case they're classified as having a high renin-sodium profile, while others have a very low renin level in the blood even when eating very little salt and so have a low renin profile.

The test is useful in three ways. First, it serves as a screening test for some of the rarer causes of high blood pressure such as a narrowing in the artery of a kidney (renovascular hypertension) or an adrenal gland tumor. Second, it provides some indication as to which type of medication is likely to work best in your case. Some types of medication lower blood pressure by blocking the effects of the renin system, and not surprisingly, they're more effective in people with a high renin profile. Third, renin is itself a risk factor for heart attacks.

Echocardiogram

Although this has been widely used by cardiologists for many years for evaluating heart disease, it's only gradually gaining acceptance as an important test in hypertension. This is a pity, because it's by far the best test for assessing whether the high blood pressure has had any effect on the heart. It's done using ultrasound, very-high-frequency sound waves that are emitted from a probe held on the skin of the chest wall, and aimed at the heart. The principle is the same as a ship's sonar: the sound waves are reflected by the tissues of the body, and the reflected waves are picked up by the probe. By displaying these signals on a monitor like a radar screen, it's possible to measure with great accuracy the thickness of the tissues, including the heart muscle, that are reflecting the sound waves. The size of the chamber, or cavity, of the heart can also be calculated. In fact, the technique is so precise that it can be used to measure the thickness of the muscle of a rat's heart (rats are commonly used as models of experimental hypertension).

When the blood pressure is high, the heart has to pump harder, and like any other muscle that's being used a lot, it enlarges. This doesn't happen straight away, but is a gradual process. One of the things that makes the echocardiogram so useful, therefore, is that it provides a sort of cumulative measure of the height of the blood pressure over the months and years preceding the test. In patients with white-coat hypertension (see Chapter 10), whose blood pressure is high only when they're in a doctor's office, the echocardiogram typically shows no signs of enlargement of the heart. But if the heart muscle is enlarged it's usually a bad omen, because prospective studies of people who've had echocardiograms have shown that the individuals with larger hearts are at much higher risk of having a heart attack than those with normal-sized hearts. If the echocardiogram does show that your heart is enlarged, therefore, it means that your blood pressure should be taken seriously, and that you will definitely need treatment.

Twenty-four-hour Blood Pressure Monitoring

The blood pressure that your doctor records in the office is generally assumed to be representative of your "true" blood pressure, by which is meant the average level over prolonged periods of time. But this isn't necessarily always the case: many people get nervous when they're seeing their doctor, so their blood pressure goes up. Twenty-four-hour (or ambulatory) monitoring is a relatively new technique that enables blood pressure to be measured outside the rather artificial setting of the doctor's office, while you go about your normal daily activities. The monitor is about the size of a Walkman radio and is worn on a belt around the waist. It's connected by a thin tube to a blood pressure cuff on the upper arm, and is relatively unobtrusive. It can be preprogrammed to take readings at regular intervals, typically every 15 to 30 minutes, throughout the day and night, and is fully automatic, which means that it pumps up the cuff, deflates it, and stores the reading in its memory. All you have to do is to hold your arm still while the reading is being taken, and also to record what you were doing at the time. At the end of the 24 hours you have the monitor disconnected, and the readings are transferred into a personal computer. Up to 100 readings may be taken, so it's possible to get a much better idea of what your true blood pressure really is.

I and my colleagues use this procedure a lot in our practice, and we find it extremely useful, particularly in patients in whom we're not sure whether their blood pressure is really high. However, there are a lot of doctors who still regard it as experimental, and many insurance companies do not reimburse for it.

THE ANKLE-ARM INDEX

A new test that physicians are starting to use for early signs of cardiovascular disease in older people is unusual in that unlike most new tests, this one is very simple. It's called the ankle-arm index, and is the ratio between the systolic blood pressure measured in the arm and in the ankle. The ankle blood pressure is measured by putting a cuff around the lower part of the calf, but instead of listening with a stethoscope, a pencil-shaped flow probe (technically known as a Doppler probe) is placed over the artery at the ankle to detect the pressure at which the blood starts to flow as the cuff pressure is reduced. For this test, the arm pressure is measured in the same way. The whole thing can be done in a few minutes.

Normally the pressures are about the same in the arm and ankle, giving a ratio of one. But in people who have diseased arteries the ankle pressure is lower than the arm pressure, such that the ankle-arm index is less than 1. You may wonder why this should be so. The reason is twofold. First, the blood pressure wave has to travel about three times the distance through the arteries to get to the ankle as to get to the el-

bow (where the arm pressure is measured), so if there is a blockage anywhere along the way there will be a falloff of pressure at the ankle; and
second, for some unknown reason atherosclerosis spares the arteries going to the arms. Thus, at a fraction of the cost of elaborate scans and angiograms, this simple test can detect atherosclerotic disease before it
starts to cause overt problems.

The importance of the test lies not so much in the information that it
provides about blockages in the circulation to the legs (which can certainly cause problems, but don't kill people), as in the fact that in people
over the age of 65 it provides a very good predictor of the risk of a stroke
or heart attack. In one study, 5 percent of elderly women who had a normal ankle-arm index died over a four-year period, while a whopping 22
percent who had an index of 0.9 or less died over the same interval.

If you're over 65 this test may be very helpful in deciding whether you
should be taking medications to lower your blood pressure or cholesterol.

TESTS FOR DIAGNOSING RARE CAUSES OF HYPERTENSION

After your initial evaluation it's possible that your doctor may suspect
that you have one of the rarer causes of hypertension, or secondary hypertension (see Chapter 14). Although these account for less than 5 percent of the total number of cases, it's important not to miss the diagnosis,
because in most instances they are curable by surgery or other procedures, so there is the possibility that you won't have to take medications
for the rest of your life. But because these conditions are relatively rare,
and the tests are expensive, most doctors order the tests only when
there's a particular reason to do so. I'll describe them briefly so you'll
know what to expect if one of them is ordered in your case.

CAPTOPRIL TEST

Captopril is a blood-pressure-lowering medication that belongs to the
class of agents known as angiotensin converting enzyme (or ACE) inhibitors, described in Chapter 22. It blocks the effects of the enzyme
that forms angiotensin, the end product of renin. When this happens,

both the amount of angiotensin in the blood and the blood pressure fall, which stimulates the kidney to release more renin. This renin response is exaggerated if one or both kidneys have a blocked artery. The captopril test is very simple to perform, and can be done in a doctor's office, with the patient sitting in a chair. At the start, a blood sample is taken for measurement of renin, and also a blood pressure reading. Then a single dose of captopril is given (by mouth), and the effects on the blood pressure are monitored. An hour later, a second blood sample is taken. When renovascular hypertension is present, the renin increases much more than in essential hypertension (the usual form).

ABDOMINAL ULTRASOUND

This test is like a radar scan of your abdomen, and has all sorts of uses. For people with high blood pressure it may be used to measure the size of the kidneys. A shrunken kidney on one side may be a clue to a blocked artery, and hence to the cause of the hypertension. It's performed by holding a probe on the abdominal wall and directing a beam of ultrasound, which is reflected by the organ being examined.

RENAL SCAN (RENOGRAM)

This test is performed to show the size and function of each kidney. It works on the principle that radioactive substances (called radioisotopes) injected into the bloodstream can be detected by a special camera (a gamma camera), which is rather like an X-ray machine. The amount of radiation used is very small. For a renal (kidney) scan an isotope that is rapidly excreted by the kidneys is used. The procedure is carried out by injecting a small dose of the isotope into an arm vein while the gamma camera takes pictures of the kidney region. As the isotope passes through the kidneys and into the urine the two kidneys "light up" on the camera images. If one kidney is not working properly (because of a blocked artery, for example) it will excrete less of the isotope than the normal kidney, and also take longer to do so. Like many other diagnostic tests, however, it's not 100 percent reliable, and may occasionally indicate an abnormality that isn't truly there; also, at times it may miss an abnormality that does exist. Its main use is for diagnosing renovascular hypertension. A more sophisticated version of it is the captopril scan, described next.

CAPTOPRIL RENAL SCAN (RENOGRAM)

Captopril is a blood-pressure-lowering medication that has a specific effect on kidney function. In normal kidneys it produces a slight increase in the rate of urine formation, but in kidneys with a blocked artery it decreases it. The captopril scan makes use of this phenomenon, and is performed by comparing two kidney scans, one done before and one after captopril is given (typically one hour after a single dose). If there is a blocked artery, the second scan should show a deterioration of function in the affected kidney when compared with the first scan. This test is relatively new, and it's still being evaluated. It's obviously more expensive and takes longer than a single scan, but when it does show a change after captopril, it is very accurate.

RENAL VEIN RENIN TEST

This is another test for diagnosing renovascular hypertension, and is performed in the radiology department of a hospital. Under local anesthesia, a flexible plastic tube (catheter) is inserted into a large vein in the groin and is pushed up inside the vein until it's at the level of the kidneys. Then, under X-ray control, the tip of the catheter is advanced into the vein draining one kidney, and a blood sample is taken for measurement of renin. Another sample is taken from the other kidney. Normally, both kidneys secrete the same amount of renin. If the artery to one kidney is obstructed, the kidney responds by making an excessive amount of renin, while the good kidney may shut off its secretion to compensate. The test is interpreted by comparing the renin levels on the two sides.

RENAL ARTERIOGRAM (ANGIOGRAM)

Of all the tests for diagnosing secondary hypertension, this is one of the few that requires admission to the hospital, although it is now beginning to be done on an outpatient basis as well. It is the most accurate way of directly visualizing the arteries to the kidneys, but because it is invasive, and not without risk, it is only performed when other less invasive tests suggest a very high probability of renal artery disease. It's performed in the radiology department. A catheter is inserted into the large artery in the groin under local anesthesia, and advanced into the aorta (the main artery of the body) as far as the level at which the arteries to the kidneys branch off. X-ray contrast medium (iodine-containing liquid that is opaque to X rays) is then injected down the catheter and outlines the renal arteries, revealing whether there's any blockage.

URINE COLLECTION FOR CATECHOLAMINES

A very rare cause of hypertension is a small tumor of the adrenal gland called a pheochromocytoma (see Chapter 14). One of the functions of the gland is to secrete epinephrine (also known as adrenaline), which belongs to a class of substances called catecholamines. The pheochromocytoma also secretes epinephrine and its sister compound norepinephrine, but in excessive quantities, which can be detected in the urine. Because the secretion is sporadic, the urine collection is made over 24 hours. The urine is collected in a plastic bottle that contains a small amount of a strong acid as a preservative for the catecholamines. Don't spill it!

CT (COMPUTERIZED TOMOGRAPHY) SCAN

CT scans are used to diagnose all sorts of diseases, and may be regarded as three-dimensional X rays, because they show the size and location of all the organs in the body. They're also very good at showing tumors. In the evaluation of hypertension their main use is the detection of adrenal gland tumors, which raise blood pressure by secreting hormones into the bloodstream. There are two main kinds: one is the pheochromocytoma, which secretes catecholamines (see above), and the other is an aldosterone-secreting tumor or adenoma. Aldosterone is another hormone that raises blood pressure. Both of these are usually benign (not cancerous), and often quite small, sometimes no bigger than a pea.

MRI (MAGNETIC RESONANCE IMAGING) SCAN

These scans provide similar information to CT scans, but work on a somewhat different principle. MRI involves placing the body into an intense magnetic field, and then taking X rays. You lie inside a large metal tube while the pictures are taken. Because of the magnetic field, it cannot be done if you have metal implanted in your body (such as a heart pacemaker or artificial hip).

SUMMARY

• Your pressure may be quite high at your first visit to your doctor; it may require several visits and a series of measurements taken away from the office to establish how high it really is.

• An extensive workup to diagnose curable but rare causes of hypertension is not routinely needed.

• The chances are that after your workup the doctor will decide that you have essential hypertension, which is treated by lifestyle changes and, if necessary, medication.

CHAPTER SEVENTEEN

MEASURING YOUR OWN BLOOD PRESSURE

A recent national survey showed that the most common reason for visiting a physician was for the measurement of blood pressure. Most people with high blood pressure do not visit their doctors more frequently than once every few weeks or months, and it is tacitly assumed that the readings taken on these occasions are representative of the level of blood pressure during the intervening period. When you think about this, it's a big assumption. Our hearts beat about 100,000 times each day, and each heartbeat produces a slightly different blood pressure. During an office visit your doctor will rarely take more than two or three readings, so if he or she sees you once every three months, these three readings will be used to represent the 9 million individual blood pressures that will occur before your next visit!

While in general this assumption holds surprisingly well, there are a number of factors that could produce a transient increase in your blood pressure at the time your doctor takes it, which could also invalidate this assumption. Let's look at some of them.

FACTORS THAT CAN RAISE THE OFFICE BLOOD PRESSURE

The White-Coat Effect. In Chapter 10, I discuss the phenomenon of white-coat hypertension. Its basis is that there are a lot of people who get nervous when they visit their doctor to have their blood pressure checked, which not surprisingly makes the blood pressure go up. Thus the doctor may record blood pressures that are as much as 20 or 30 mm

Hg higher than at other times. To some extent, this wears off as you become more familiar with your doctor and the setting in which he or she works, but I have patients whom I have been following for ten years who still show this phenomenon unabated. Most people who are labeled as being hypertensive on the basis of their clinic or office blood pressure have home blood pressures that are lower than the office pressures.

Food and Drink. Contrary to what you might think, eating a Chinese meal the night before you have your blood pressure checked is unlikely to affect it very much. Even infusing salt solution directly into the veins of hypertensive subjects has a negligible immediate effect on their blood pressure. Several studies have investigated the effects of different types of meals on blood pressure, and most have found that there is little change, except in older people, who may experience quite a large fall in pressure about 40 minutes after eating. Drinking coffee, on the other hand, can raise pressure, as described in more detail in Chapter 7.

Smoking. If you smoke just before your blood pressure is measured, it may be 5 mm Hg higher than it would have been otherwise. And the combination of drinking a cup of coffee and smoking a cigarette can produce an even bigger increase that lasts for two hours or more.

Your Mood. If you've had a bad day at work, you couldn't find a parking spot for your car, and then the doctor keeps you waiting, it won't be surprising if your pressure is found to be high.

Talking. It is not widely appreciated, even by many doctors, that talking can produce a substantial increase of blood pressure. This phenomenon has been described by Dr. James Lynch, who put an automatic monitor on a patient, and observed that when the patient was sitting quietly he had a blood pressure of 148/78, but when he started to talk it went up to 162/91. So if your doctor is taking a series of blood pressure measurements, don't ask what the pressure was after each reading.

The Time of Day. Blood pressure tends to be a little higher in the morning than in the afternoon or evening, although this pattern varies from one person to another. There's not usually a big difference unless you're taking medications, in which case the length of time since you took your last pill may make a big difference.

The Season of the Year. In temperate climates, where there are large temperature differences between summer and winter, blood pressure tends to be about 5 mm Hg higher in the winter than in the summer.

THE ADVANTAGES OF SELF-MONITORING

All except the last of these problems can in principle be avoided by supplementing the readings taken in the doctor's office by readings taken outside it. This has two advantages: First, it increases the total number of readings available from which to estimate the overall or average level of blood pressure, which is what is thought to be ultimately important in determining its consequences. Everyone gets the occasional high reading, and the significance (or lack of significance) of these can best be appreciated if there are a large number of other readings, so that they can be put into their proper perspective. When patients first start taking their blood pressure, they are frequently astonished at how variable it is, and no less frequently worried about the few readings that seem excessively high.

The second advantage of measuring your own blood pressure is that it avoids the potentially distorting influence of the doctor's office, or the white-coat effect. This means that in the majority of patients the pressure recorded at home is substantially lower than that in the doctor's office. It may still be high, but when it's definitely normal (for example, below 135/85 mm Hg), it's highly questionable whether you should start taking medications.

THE DISADVANTAGES OF HOME MONITORING

Despite the undoubted benefits of home monitoring, it has to be admitted that it's not for everyone. Most people actually find it reassuring to learn that their blood pressure at home is not as high as in the doctor's office, but there is a minority who get panicky at the thought of putting a blood pressure cuff on themselves, and can even generate their own white-coat syndrome, whereby the anxiety associated with taking blood pressure can make it go up.

HOW TO MEASURE YOUR BLOOD PRESSURE

Measuring your own pressure is neither expensive nor difficult, but there are some potential pitfalls. First is the question of equipment. We routinely recommend what is in fact the simplest and cheapest device, known as an aneroid sphygmomanometer. This consists of a blood pressure cuff that goes around your arm, connected by a rubber tube to a dial that registers the pressure. You also need a stethoscope. The whole thing costs about $30, which may be less than the cost of a doctor's visit. Some of the currently available models (recently reviewed by *Consumer Reports* magazine) are listed in Table 17.1. All of them include a stethoscope, which in most cases is attached to the cuff. This makes the measurement of blood pressure much easier.

The cuff is put on your nondominant arm, that is, your left arm if you're right-handed. The ones that are easiest to use have a metal buckle or D-ring, around which you can loop the loose end of the cuff, to pull it tight on the Velcro fastener. (All the models listed in the table have this.) Before you pump up the cuff, it should be just tight enough to fit snugly around your arm, without actually squeezing it. It's important to position the cuff correctly, which is on your upper arm just above the elbow joint. The rubber bag inside the cuff does not occupy its entire length, and should be located with the middle of the bag over the artery, which it will occlude when inflated. With most cuffs this means positioning the cuff so that the tubes are located a little toward the inner side of your arm.

The cuff is inflated by screwing tight the knob by the bulb, and then pumping up the bulb to a pressure of about 200 mm Hg, or to well above your systolic pressure. You then unscrew the knob a little, to let air gradually out of the cuff. The ideal rate of deflation is about 2 or 3 mm Hg per second (or about 2 or 3 mm Hg per thud, when you start hearing the sounds).

The stethoscope is placed just below the edge of the cuff over the artery. To find the right position you should be able to feel the pulsations of the artery by pressing two fingers lightly over the front of your elbow crease, at the bottom end of your biceps muscle.

If you've pumped up the cuff high enough, you should hear nothing at first, but as you deflate it you'll start to hear the *Korotkoff sounds*, which are dull thuds in time with your heartbeats. They are caused by the artery opening and shutting, and by blood spurting through the narrowed portion. The first sound that you hear gives you the systolic pressure. As you deflate the cuff further, the sounds get louder, then more muffled, and then start to fade out. The last sound you hear (technically known as phase 5 of the Korotkoff sounds) gives you the diastolic pressure. Some people advocate taking the muffling (or phase 4) of the sounds just before they disappear, but this is much less reliable, and I do not recommend it.

Table 17.1. Home Blood Pressure Monitors

ANEROID (NONELECTRONIC) DEVICES

NAME	PRICE	SI*	ACCURACY	COMMENTS
Marshall 104	$29	No	Good	Top-rated by CR
Omron HEM-18	$30	No	Good	Top-rated by CR
Walgreen's 2001	$20	No	Good	
Lumiscope 100-02	$30	No	Good	
Sunmark 100	$22	No	Good	
Sunbeam 7627-10	$31	No	Good	Stethoscope not attached to cuff

ELECTRONIC DEVICES

NAME	PRICE	SI*	ACCURACY	COMMENTS
Omron HEM-704C	$130	Yes	Good	Top-rated by CR
Sunbeam 7621	$ 62	No	Good	Top-rated by CR
Sunbeam 7650	$115	Yes	Good	Top-rated by CR
Lumiscope 1081	$100	Yes	Fair	
Marshall 91	$118	Yes	Fair	
AND UA-701	$ 45	No	Good	
Omron HEM-713C	$ 90	Yes	Fair	
Sunmark 144	$ 48	No	Fair	
Omron HEM-413C	$ 52	No	Fair	
Walgreen's 80WA	$ 40	No	Fair	
Marshall 80	$ 60	No	Fair	
Lumiscope 1065	$ 60	No	Fair	
AND UA-731	$ 79	Yes	Poor	
Radio Shack 63663	$ 50	No	Poor	
Lumiscope 1060	$ 60	No	Poor	

*SI = self-inflating.

Source: Adapted from *Consumer Reports,* May 1992.

How Reliable Are the Electronic Monitors?

Virtually any drugstore will offer a variety of automatic or semiautomatic blood pressure monitors. You don't need a stethoscope, and all you have to do is put on the cuff, switch the machine on, and let it take a reading, which it will display on a digital readout, together with your heart rate. It sounds good, doesn't it?

There is no doubt that these devices have their uses, particularly for people who have a hearing problem, or who may lack the manual dexterity to put on and pump up a cuff with one hand. They have one major drawback, however—they are often not very accurate. The fact that a machine displays a number for your blood pressure doesn't necessarily mean that it's the right number. Some years ago we performed a study in which we checked the accuracy of 11 different types of monitors against readings taken simultaneously by a trained observer using a conventional sphygmomanometer and stethoscope, and found that some of the electronic monitors were in error by as much as 16 mm Hg. More recently, *Consumer Reports* magazine (May 1992) evaluated 6 aneroid and 15 electronic devices, and got more encouraging results. These are noted in Table 17.1. Unfortunately, the criteria by which the monitors were tested were not described, and most of these newer monitors have not been tested in a scientifically rigorous way. One exception is the Omron HEM-704C, which has been shown to be accurate.

WHAT IF I NEED A LARGE CUFF?

If your doctor tells you that you need a large cuff to measure your blood pressure accurately (because you either are overweight or have a very well-developed biceps muscle), this could pose a problem with some of the home monitors. All of them come with the standard cuff size, but not all can be used with a large cuff. If you get an aneroid device, it is very easy to replace the standard cuff with a large cuff, which you can buy at any good drugstore for about $25. If you buy an electronic one, replacing the standard cuff may be more of a problem, because it may not be easy to unplug and replace the cuff. With some of the models listed in the table (Lumiscope 1081 and 1065, Marshall 80 and 91, and AND UA-701) you can substitute a large cuff for an additional cost of $30 to $35.

HOW MUCH DO HOME MONITORS COST?

Home monitors are very cost-effective, and the actual cost ranges from about $30 to $150. The nonelectronic (aneroid) devices cost as little as $30, the manually inflated electronic ones about $40 to $60, and the self-inflating ones about $90 to $130.

FINGER MONITORS

Without any doubt, the simplest monitors available are ones that take your blood pressure from a finger. All you have to do is stick your finger through a plastic ring, which contains a miniature cuff, and press the button. This makes the monitor inflate and deflate the cuff, and then display the reading. It sounds attractive, but unfortunately the technique is not very reliable. It's important to keep your finger at the level of your heart (in the "salute the flag" position); otherwise the monitors will give falsely high or low readings. Even if you do this, however, the monitors are not very accurate. We do not recommend them for our patients, and *Consumer Reports* came to the same conclusion.

How Often Should Readings Be Taken?

When you've taken the trouble to get out your blood pressure monitor and set it up, it makes sense to take more than one reading. A lot of people find that, even when taking their own blood pressure, the first reading is higher than subsequent ones (the same as happens when a doctor is taking your pressure), so I usually recommend taking a series of two or three readings on each occasion. It's also a good idea to take readings at different times of day (particularly if you're taking medications), in case there's a difference between morning and evening values.

How many days a week you take your pressure depends to a large extent on where you are in your treatment program. If you're in the early stages, when it's still not clear whether you need to start taking medication, it's helpful to take readings relatively frequently (for example, three or four times a week for at least two weeks). When you're just starting on medication, or when the dose has been changed, frequent readings are again advisable. But if you're on a stable dose and your pressure is controlled, once or twice a month may be all that is needed.

What Is an Acceptable Level of Home Blood Pressure?

Ideally, the average level of home blood pressure should be a bit lower than the acceptable levels of clinic blood pressure—for example, below 135 to 140 mm Hg for systolic pressure, and 85 to 90 for diastolic. In older patients I would be quite happy with higher values for the systolic pressure, of up to 160 mm Hg.

SUMMARY

• Measuring your own blood pressure has a lot of advantages: it enables you to get a series of readings taken over several days or weeks, to establish a baseline level free from the anxiety-provoking influence of the doctor's office.

• It's also a very good way to monitor your response to treatment.

• Devices for measuring your pressure are cheap and easy to use; you can get either an aneroid device or an approved electronic one, but in either case you should have your doctor check the device and your technique.

• Don't get a finger monitor.

• Discuss with your doctor how often you should be taking readings, and then keep a written record of the numbers.

PART TWO

WHAT YOU CAN DO ABOUT HIGH BLOOD PRESSURE: CHANGING YOUR BEHAVIOR—THE STAIRCASE TO SUCCESS

All of us are creatures of habit and have our daily rituals, which we follow without thinking. We're also very resistant to changing these rituals, as we slide along the groove of our lives. Since high blood pressure is a condition that does not go away by itself, most of the behavioral changes that are recommended for dealing with it need to be permanent and to become part of your daily ritual. Jolting yourself from one groove to another is not easy, but once you've done it, these changes can become part of your new ritual.

When people do change their behavior, they usually go through a series of stages that may be likened to going up a staircase. Progress is not always smooth, and you may go back a step as well as forward. The stages have been characterized by Dr. James Prochaska, a psychologist at the University of Rhode Island, and are based on interviews with people who succeeded in making these changes. They are as follows.

1. *Precontemplation.* At this stage you have no plans to make any changes, either because you are unaware of the consequences of your behavior, or because you are unconvinced of the benefits of change, or your ability to do it.
2. *Contemplation* is the stage at which you seriously plan to change your behavior in the next six months, but are not yet ready to actually do it.
3. *Preparation.* By now you are convinced that you are going to make a change, and are starting to do something, such as cutting down on the number of cigarettes you smoke. This stage typically lasts from one to six months.
4. *Action* is the stage when you are actually making the changes. This

is the high-stakes period, when you either succeed or don't. It lasts for up to six months.

5. *Maintenance.* If you make it to this stage, you're just about home. You've quit your habit, although there's still a chance that you could relapse to the bad old ways. This stage can last for up to five years.

6. *Termination.* By now, you're home and dry, and immune to temptation.

WILL I LIVE LONGER IF I CHANGE MY BEHAVIOR?

Several studies have attempted to estimate the changes in life expectancy that would occur as a result of changing behavior patterns that are associated with an increased risk of heart disease. The ones that have received the most attention are going on a low-fat diet and quitting smoking. The studies have used computer modeling techniques, and are based on what is known about the relationships between blood cholesterol, smoking habits, and heart disease. The results may surprise you.

A recent example was published by Dr. Steven Grover and his colleagues from Montreal. They calculated the change in life expectancy of Canadians who followed either the Step One or Step Two diet of the American Heart Association (described in Chapter 18), and who quit smoking (if they smoked). The results are shown in Table II.1. The Step One diet is a moderate low-fat diet; the Step Two diet is more rigorous.

Table II.1. Estimated Increases in Life Expectancy as a Result of Adopting a Low-Fat Diet or Quitting Smoking

| | | INCREASE IN LIFE EXPECTANCY | | |
SEX	AGE	DIET 1	DIET 2	STOP SMOKING
Male	30–39	3 months	5 months	4 years
	40–49	4 months	5 months	4 years
	50–59	2 months	3 months	4 years
	60–69	3 weeks	1 month	3 years
	70–79	2 weeks	3 weeks	3 years
Female	30–39	3 weeks	1 month	4 years
	40–49	3 weeks	2 months	4 years
	50–59	3 weeks	1 month	3 years
	60–69	2 weeks	3 weeks	3 years
	70–79	4 days	2 weeks	3 years

Source: Grover & colleagues: *Archives of Internal Medicine,* 1994.

There are several points to make from this table. The first, of course, is the paltry effect of the low-fat diets. To make a radical change in your diet and live a few months longer may not be worth the effort. Actually, even these figures are very optimistic, because they assume that the Step One diet will lower cholesterol by 17 mg/dl in men and 5 in women, changes that are much bigger than have been observed in practice. Another point is the much greater benefit derived from quitting smoking. You'll also notice that the benefits are greatest in middle-aged men and are less in women and the elderly.

One of the reasons the benefits appear so small is that they are averages for the population as a whole, and they would be greater in people who are at higher risk to begin with, as shown in Table II.2, which is from another study using the same type of procedure.

Table II.2. Estimated Increases in Life Expectancy from Risk Modification for 35-Year-Old Men at Different Levels of Initial Risk

INTERVENTION	INCREASE IN LIFE EXPECTANCY
Reduce cholesterol to 200 mg/dl	
Initial level 200–239	6 months
Initial level 240–299	1–2 years
Initial level over 300	4 years
Reduce cigarettes smoked	
By 50%	1–2 years
Quit	3–4 years
Reduce diastolic blood pressure to 88 mm Hg	
Initial level 90–94	1 year
Initial level 95–104	2 years
Initial level over 105	5 years
Reduce weight to ideal weight	
Initially 0%–30% overweight	6 months
Initially more than 30% overweight	1–2 years

Source: Tsevat & colleagues: *Circulation*, 1991.

CHAPTER EIGHTEEN

CHANGING YOUR DIET

Changing your diet may not necessarily cure your high blood pressure, but there is a lot that can affect your general state of health one way or the other. Since heart disease is the major risk associated with high blood pressure, it makes sense to choose a diet that minimizes your risk of this, as well as lowering your blood pressure. The focus should be on a diet that is generally healthy, rather than on one that is exclusively focused on blood pressure. Just because you have high blood pressure it does not mean that you are going to have a stroke or a heart attack, nor does it make you immune from getting cancer.

The conventional dietary recommendation for people with high blood pressure is to restrict fat and salt. Official bodies such as the American Heart Association and the National Cholesterol Education Program have mounted national campaigns to encourage the general public, whether hypertensive or not, to go on a low-fat diet, and the U.S. Department of Agriculture has promulgated a "Food Guide Pyramid" to show us how to achieve these goals. As we'll see, however, simply restricting your fat intake is not the only way to go, and there is increasing evidence that substituting "good fat" (monounsaturated fatty acids) for "bad fat" (saturated fatty acids), as in the Mediterranean diet, not only is much more palatable, but may also be more effective.

In this chapter I will review both types of approach, and you can decide which one is for you.

THE AMERICAN HEART ASSOCIATION LOW-FAT DIETS

The American Heart Association has come up with two general types of diet aimed at lowering blood cholesterol levels. The "Step One" diet is more moderate, and the "Step Two" is for people with high cholesterol and known cardiovascular disease. The overall guidelines, and a comparison with the typical American diet, are shown in Table 18.1. Cookbooks based on these diets are published by the AHA, and are listed at the end of this chapter.

Table 18.1. AHA Diets Compared with the Typical American Diet

Nutrient*	Typical U.S. Diet	AHA Step 1 Diet	AHA Step 2 Diet
Total fat	35%–40%	Below 30%	Below 30%
Saturated fat	15%–20%	Below 10%	Below 7%
Polyunsaturated fat	7%	Up to 10%	Up to 10%
Monounsaturated fat	15%	10%–15%	10%–15%
Carbohydrate	47%	50%–60%	50%–60%
Protein	16%	10%–20%	10%–20%
Cholesterol	450 mg	Below 300 mg	Below 200 mg

*The different types of fats are described in Chapter 2.

These dietary recommendations have been advocated in a somewhat different form as the USDA Food Guide Pyramid, described next.

THE USDA FOOD GUIDE PYRAMID AND THE SIX FOOD GROUPS

A few years ago the U.S. Department of Agriculture introduced the "Food Guide Pyramid" to visually demonstrate the recommended proportions of the six major food groups in the ideal diet. This is shown in Figure 18.1. Groups 1 and 2 are foods rich in fats; they come at the tip of the pyramid, and are hence supposed to be eaten "sparingly." Group 3 is foods rich in protein, while Groups 4 through 6 are carbohydrates, which contribute the bulk of the calories, and hence are at the base of the pyramid.

Group 1: Fats, Oils, and Sweets (Use sparingly)

Items in this group come at the top of the pyramid because they tend to be high in fats and high in calories. They include butter, margarine, desserts, candies, salad dressings, and oils. They are supposed to be kept to a minimum.

Figure 18.1.   **USDA FOOD GUIDE PYRAMID**

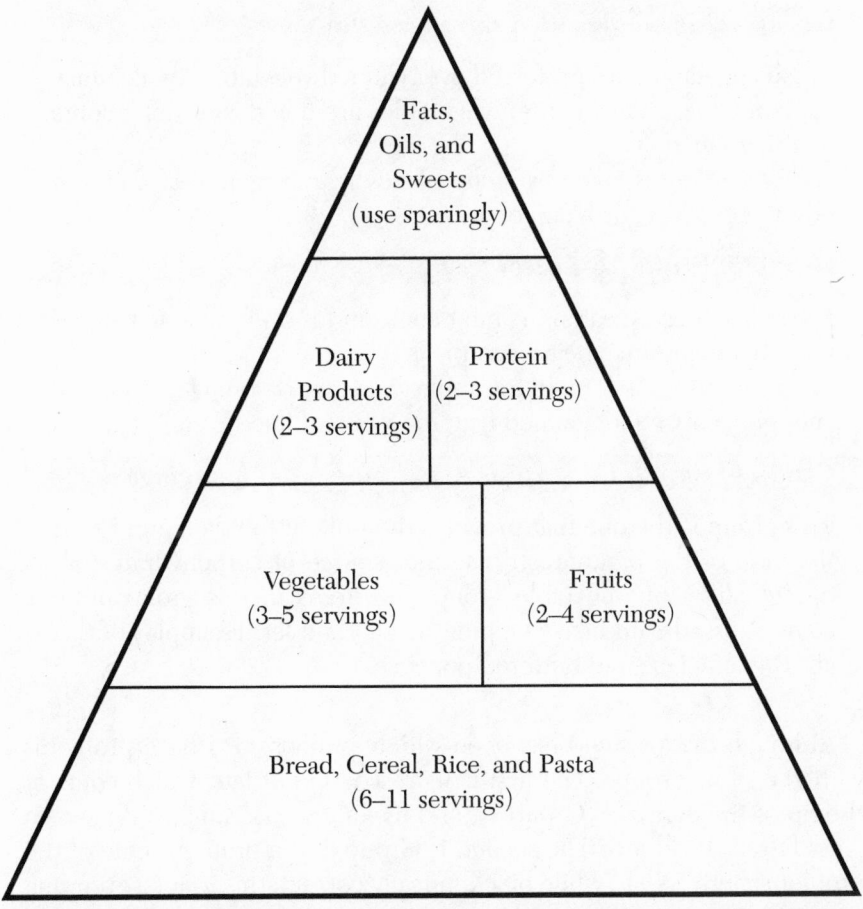

Fats,
Oils, and
Sweets
(use sparingly)

Dairy
Products
(2–3 servings)

Protein
(2–3 servings)

Vegetables
(3–5 servings)

Fruits
(2–4 servings)

Bread, Cereal, Rice, and Pasta
(6–11 servings)

Group 2: Milk, Yogurt, and Cheese (2–3 servings a day)

This group is a major source of calcium, but also tends to be high in saturated fat. Nevertheless, all three are available in low-fat forms.

One serving is 1 cup of milk or yogurt, 1½ ounces of natural cheese, or 2 ounces of processed cheese.

Group 3: Meat, Poultry, Fish, Dry Beans, Eggs, and Nuts (2–3 servings a day)

This group provides protein, which you don't have to get from meat. Egg whites are an excellent source, as of course is fish, and you can also substitute dried beans, peas, lentils, or tofu.

One serving is 2 to 3 ounces of cooked meat, poultry, or fish; 1½ cups of beans; or 2 egg whites.

Group 4: Vegetables (3–5 servings a day)

Fresh vegetables are preferred over canned vegetables (which may contain a lot of salt). Frozen vegetables are fine if they don't come in a rich sauce.

One serving is taken as 1 cup of raw leafy vegetables, ½ cup of other vegetables, or ¾ cup of juice.

Group 5: Fruits (2–4 servings a day)

Fresh fruit can be eaten in abundance, and is preferable to canned fruit that comes in a heavy syrup.

One serving is 1 medium apple, banana, or orange; ½ cup of chopped, cooked, or canned fruit; or ¾ cup of juice.

Group 6: Bread, Cereal, Rice, and Pasta (6–11 servings a day)

This group is the one that provides the bulk of the diet, and forms the base of the pyramid. It's another source of carbohydrates, although, like the vegetable group, the items in this group often come dressed with heavy helpings of salt and fat. Examples of this are Ritz crackers and buttered popcorn.

Although this pyramid has been widely publicized, I have problems with two of its groups. The first is its restriction of fats, which come at the tip of the pyramid (Group 1), and its failure to distinguish between good fats and bad fats. The second is Group 3, the proteins. One of the problems here is that, while biochemically correct, this is not a grouping that fits with any natural culinary grouping. When we're deciding what to eat we may certainly choose between meat, poultry, or fish, but I think that if my wife asked me whether I'd prefer meat, dry beans, or nuts for dinner I would seriously question her sanity. And since you are supposed to be able to make your choices within each group, the pyramid implies that it is perfectly acceptable to eat three servings of red meat every day (a total of 9 ounces), or in other words you can eat steak at breakfast, lunch, and dinner, and stay healthy!

The new Mediterranean Food Pyramid, described on the next few pages, gets around both of these problems.

WHY LOW-FAT DIETS MAY NOT BE THE ANSWER

The American Heart Association's manual entitled *Dietary Treatment of Hypercholesterolemia* states that most people usually reach their blood cholesterol–lowering goal with the Step One diet within three months. In my experience, many patients are disappointed by the small changes in blood cholesterol that take place after changing their diet; they are not alone. Some years ago Dr. Larry Ramsay, an English physician, surveyed the medical literature for reports of the effectiveness of the Step One and Step Two diets. For the Step One diet the fall of total blood cholesterol ranged from 0 to 4 percent, and for the more rigorous Step Two diet from 6 to 15 percent. Since he published his survey the results of another large study have been published, with even more dismal changes. This showed that the Step Two diet lowered total and LDL cholesterol by only 5 percent, but that it also lowered HDL by the same amount, so the ratio of good to bad cholesterol was unchanged.

Dr. Ramsay concluded from this survey that the official recommendations that most people with high cholesterol levels can control them with diet alone are "totally unrealistic," and I agree with him. This does not mean to say that a low-fat diet is not worth trying, because you may be one of the lucky ones who responds very well, but it does mean that you shouldn't feel guilty if it doesn't seem to be working. The same thing applies to the effects of a low-salt diet on blood pressure, of course.

Even if the goals of the diet are successfully achieved there are still problems with the AHA low-fat diet. One is that it lowers the HDL (good) cholesterol, which means that the beneficial effects on atherosclerosis are less than they would be if the HDL was maintained or raised. One of the advantages of eating olive oil (monounsaturated fat) over other types of oil (polyunsaturated fat) is that it lowers total cholesterol without also lowering HDL. Another limitation of this diet is that it makes no recommendation to increase the intake of monounsaturated fats; if you follow it strictly, your intake will go down rather than up. Canola oil is one of the recommended cooking oils, and as we saw in Chapter 4, there are still concerns about its safety. Finally, there is little attention paid to the dangers of *trans*–fatty acids, which are found in hydrogenated vegetable oils and margarines (see also Chapter 4).

THE ADVANTAGES OF THE MEDITERRANEAN DIET

As we saw in Chapter 4, studies of different populations around the world have shown that heart disease tends to be commoner in countries where people traditionally eat a lot of fat, with some notable exceptions, particularly the French and the Greeks. In both cases the incidence of heart disease is low, despite the fact that their consumption of fat is high. The critical factor appears to be not how much fat you eat, but what sort. What distinguishes the diets of the French, Greeks, and other Mediterranean peoples such as the Italians is that they get their fat as monounsaturated fat (MUFA), because their cuisine is based on olive oil. Other features of the Mediterranean diet are a high intake of fruits and vegetables, and a relatively low meat consumption. Complex carbohydrates are a major component, in the form of whole-grain breads, grains, and cereals.

The virtues of the Mediterranean diet are only now beginning to be appreciated. In 1991, two of the leading experts in the relationships between nutrition and disease, Drs. Frank Sacks and Walter Willett, wrote an editorial in the influential *New England Journal of Medicine* espousing its benefits. They pointed out that not all fat is alike, and that the chief culprit is saturated, or "land-mammal," fat. They questioned the conventional wisdom of replacing land-mammal fat with carbohydrate, because this tends to lower HDL cholesterol as well as LDL. In 1993 they organized a conference entitled "Traditional Diets of the Mediterranean" under the auspices of the Harvard School of Public Health, which brought together a group of international experts to discuss the subject. One of the products of this meeting was an alternative to the USDA Food Guide Pyramid, which is shown in Figure 18.2.

THE MEDITERRANEAN FOOD PYRAMID

The basis of this is the traditional Mediterranean diet that was current in about 1960, at which time the Mediterranean populations had some of the lowest rates of chronic disease and the longest life expectancies, despite relatively limited access to medical care. It is substantially different from the USDA pyramid and is much simpler to implement, because it is divided into three sections. The major difference is that it is not a low-fat diet, because it substitutes monounsaturated fat (olive oil) for satu-

Figure 18.2. **MEDITERRANEAN FOOD PYRAMID**

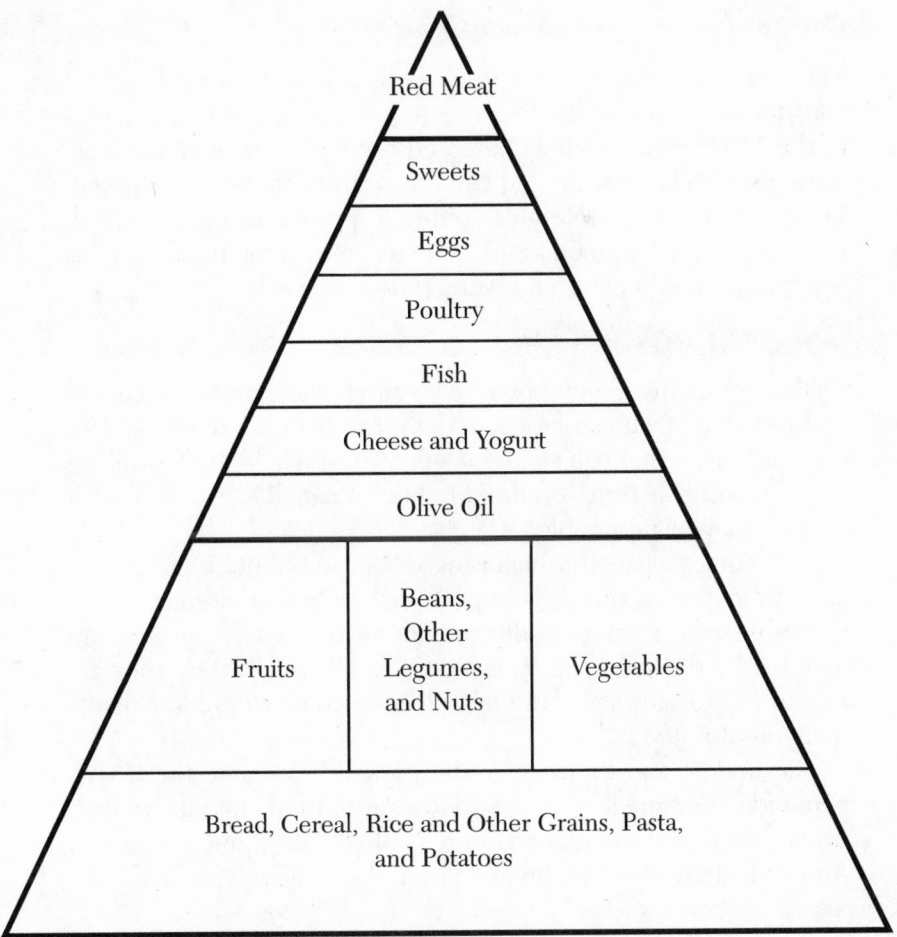

rated fat. As with the USDA pyramid, the foods at the top should be consumed less frequently than the ones at the bottom, which form the basis of the diet. They are divided into three categories.

Category One: A Few Times per Month

The sole occupant of the apex of the pyramid is red meat. A lot of evidence now suggests that a high meat intake is associated not only with heart disease but also with colon and prostate cancers. Furthermore, all the nutrients found in meat can be obtained from other sources.

Category Two: A Few Times per Week

This group is a mixed bag. At the top (which means least frequent consumption) are sweets. Desserts (other than fruit) are not a part of the Mediterranean diet, and need not be a part of yours. Next are eggs, which are restricted because of their cholesterol content. Poultry, which is a preferable source of protein to red meat, follows, but it is not as good as fish, which comes at the bottom of this group, and should be eaten several times per week.

Category Three: Every Day

At the top of this group come dairy products (principally cheese and yogurt), which can be taken daily, but in small amounts. This does not mean that you should drink a lot of whole milk (drinking milk is not a feature of the Mediterranean diet), and low-fat cheeses may be preferable.

Next comes olive oil, which is used instead of butter, margarine, and other cooking oils. It is important to note that although other vegetable oils, such as safflower and soybean oils, are recommended by the American Heart Association and USDA, they are rich in polyunsaturated fat. Only olive oil contains predominantly monounsaturated fat.

The middle and the base of the pyramid resemble the USDA pyramid in that the foods are carbohydrates. In the middle we have fruits, beans and nuts (good sources of protein), and vegetables. And at the base there are breads, pasta, rice, other grains, and potatoes.

WHICH TYPE OF COOKING OIL SHOULD I USE?

There are at the present time two schools of thought about what the preferred type of cooking oil should be. According to the NCEP and AHA all should be used sparingly, and the best are those that are rich in polyunsaturated fats (safflower, sunflower, and corn oil). The alternative viewpoint, to which I subscribe, is that olive oil is the best. There are several reasons for this. First, there is increasing evidence that monounsaturated fats are beneficial to the heart, and olive oil has the highest content (see Table 18.2). Second, there is a huge amount of epidemiological evidence to show that people who eat an olive oil–based diet live longer and healthier lives. There are no populations that have traditionally lived on safflower or sunflower oil, and we simply have no idea as to the long-term consequences of diets based on their use. In Chapter 4, I discussed some of the evidence that shows that canola oil (another supposedly "healthy" oil) causes heart damage. Third, olive oil tastes good, and is the basis of an enormously rich culinary tradition. Nothing else comes close.

The only disadvantage that I can see to olive oil is its greater cost than the others' (see Table 18.2). However, if you regard it as a medicine as well as a food, it's really dirt cheap.

Table 18.2. Fat Content and Cost of Different Cooking Oils
(Amounts of fats are shown as grams in one tablespoon of oil)

Type	Polyunsaturated Fat	Saturated Fat	Monounsaturated Fat	Cost (per 24 oz.)
Polyunsaturated oils				
Safflower oil	10.1	1.2	1.6	$2.50
Sunflower oil	8.9	1.4	2.7	$2.20
Corn oil	8.0	1.7	3.3	$1.90
Soybean oil	7.9	2.0	3.2	$3.00
Monounsaturated oils				
Canola oil	4.5	0.8	8.7	$2.20
Peanut oil	4.3	2.3	6.2	$3.70
Olive oil	1.1	1.8	9.9	$6.00–$12.00

USING THE NEW FOOD LABELING SYSTEM

In 1990 Congress passed a law requiring the Food and Drug Administration to develop a new system of food labeling, to be used on virtually every container of food that is sold. The goal was to provide standardized and intelligible labels showing the amounts of major nutrients, and also to limit health claims of being "low fat" or having "less sodium." After considerable infighting between the FDA and the Department of

Agriculture (which is responsible for the labeling of meat products, and subjected to lobbying by the meat industry), an agreement was reached for a unified and simplified system, which was introduced in May 1994.

The new labels describe the total calories, calories from fat, and the amounts of fat, saturated fat, cholesterol, fiber, complex carbohydrates, sugars, protein, sodium, vitamins A and C, calcium, and iron. They do not, unfortunately, say how much *trans*–fatty acid is present (as described in Chapter 4, such acids are now thought to be important in causing heart disease), but they do say if partially hydrogenated vegetable oils are included, and this is a clue to the presence of *trans*–fatty acids.

What makes the new labels so much easier to read than the earlier forms is that in addition to telling you what the actual amount of each nutrient is in each portion, they also tell you what the percentage of the recommended daily total is. For most of us, being informed that a food item contains 28 percent of the recommended total of sodium rather than that it has 660 milligrams makes much more sense. The problem here is that some assumptions have to be made as to what the daily total should be. This depends on who you are: the average caloric intake may be about 2,500 calories for men under the age of 50, while women in their thirties and forties consume only 1,600 calories on average.

The labels are based on a 2,000-calorie diet, but also suggest daily intakes based on a diet of 2,500 calories. For these two levels, the recommended totals of the most relevant nutrients are as shown in Table 18.3.

Table 18.3. FDA Recommendations for Normal Daily Intakes of Major Nutrients

Nutrient	2,000-Calorie Diet	2,500-Calorie Diet
Total fat	Less than 65 g	80 g
Saturated fat	Less than 20 g	25 g
Cholesterol	Less than 300 mg	300 mg
Sodium	Less than 2,400 mg	2,400 mg
Carbohydrate	300 g	375 g
Fiber	25 g	30 g

Notice that for fat, carbohydrate, and fiber, the recommended total is different depending on your overall caloric needs, while for sodium and cholesterol they are the same. What this means in practice is that if you are a petite woman you should cut the 2,000-calorie recommendations for fat, carbohydrate, and fiber by about one third, while if you're a six-foot-tall man you can go by the 2,500-calorie recommendations.

Here are some points to be aware of to help you interpret the labels:

- Serving Size: Most of us consume more than the serving size shown on the label.
- Low Calorie: These foods contain fewer than 40 calories per serving.
- Reduced Calorie: These foods contain one-third fewer calories than the standard product.
- Low Sodium: The total sodium content is less than 140 mg.
- Lite or Light: This has no legal definition, and may mean light in color, calories, or salt content.
- Low Fat: Less than 3 grams per serving.
- Low Saturated Fat: Less than 1 gram per serving.
- Low Cholesterol: Less than 20 milligrams of cholesterol and 2 grams of saturated fat per serving.
- Fat Free: Less than half a gram of fat per serving.

HOW ACCURATE ARE THE FOOD LABELS?

The fact that there is now a law regulating the use of phrases such as "low fat" and "low calorie" may be a two-edged sword, and give you a false sense of security when you buy such foods. In New York City stores that sell machine-dispensed frozen desserts with enticing names such as Skimpy Treat and Slender Delight are required to post their nutritional content. *New York* magazine recently sent samples of soft-serve frozen desserts and muffins to laboratories that analyzed the actual food contents. Almost without exception, the posted claims bore little resemblance to the actual contents. One brand of peanut butter–flavored frozen yogurt was claimed to contain 47 calories and zero fat, and actually had 323 calories and 12.5 grams of fat. A honey-bran muffin with apples and raisins that was advertised as an "All Natural, No Sugar Added Bran Muffin" was rated by *New York* as a "muffin from hell," since the analysis showed that it contained 1,000 calories and 49 grams of fat, more than in five McDonald's hamburgers.

Part of the discrepancy comes from the fact that many of the posted contents were based on sample sizes so small that they wouldn't satisfy a small child, let alone an adult. More important, although the laws have been passed, there are no diet police to see that the claims are accurate. You're probably relatively safe with foods made by large manufacturers such as Nabisco (the nutritional claim for their SnackWell's devil's food fat-free cookie was found to be accurate by *New York*), but even this may not always be true. *New York* also analyzed an individually wrapped fat-free chocolate crunch cake made by Entenmann's (a subsidiary of General Foods): while the fat-free claim was upheld (the actual content being 0.4 grams), the actual calorie content was 266 calories, whereas the claimed content was 180. When an official from the company was questioned on this point, her reply was "the philosophy of Entenmann's is to provide value—to give more than the weight on the label, rather than less."

The moral here is clear: be suspicious of the claims of desserts and baked goods, particularly if they are from small manufacturers. They are generally bad news, and the foods often contain large amounts of *trans*–fatty acids, which are not described by the food labels. Let the dieter beware!

KNOWING WHERE THE SALT COMES FROM

The first step in reducing your salt intake is finding out where the salt is coming from. In principle, salt can get into your food in five ways (see Table 18.4): what's in the raw ingredients, what's added during processing, what you add during cooking, and what you add at the table; there's also some salt in your drinking water, although this is usually trivial. For most of us, the salt we add at the table is relatively unimportant, so merely throwing out the salt shaker is not going to be enough to make an impact. More than three quarters of our salt comes from processed foods, which are more than half the food we eat. They include not only food that comes in a box or a can, but also bread and cheese.

Table 18.4. Where Our Salt Comes From

Processing	77%
Raw ingredients	12%
Added at table	6%
Cooking	5%
Water	Less than 1%

The key to success is choosing foods that are low in sodium to begin with, and this requires a certain amount of knowledge. Fortunately, the new food labeling system (see above) makes this a lot easier. The new labels give the sodium content in milligrams.

Working out your salt intake means that you are going to have to read food labels very carefully. You are no doubt well aware that potato chips, pretzels, and canned soups have a lot of salt, but most of the salt we eat is hidden in processed foods. It's put in partly for the flavor, but also for other reasons. In baked goods it's included as baking soda because it makes a better dough. In processed meats it's added as a preservative and to improve the texture.

What this means in practice is that you will need to eat less processed foods and to substitute fresh fruit and vegetables. A 3½-ounce serving of fresh garden peas contains only 2 milligrams of sodium, but the same amount of canned peas has 236 milligrams. The process of canning incidentally also tends to remove much of the potassium, so that's another reason for choosing fresh vegetables. There are a few vegetables that do contain salt without any processing; examples are celery, kale, spinach, and turnips.

Cereals and bread also contain salt (see Table 18.5 for some examples). Again, you have to read the labels: Old Fashioned Quaker Oats have none, Kellogg's All-Bran has 140 milligrams per ounce, and Kellogg's Corn Flakes 320 (an ounce of Planter's Cocktail Peanuts has only 132 mg). And two slices of Pepperidge Farm White Bread have more sodium (234 mg) than a 1-ounce bag of potato chips (191 mg).

Even sweets may have a lot of salt: half a cup of Jell-O Chocolate Flavor Instant Pudding and Pie Filling has 404 milligrams (more than three slices of Oscar Mayer bacon, which have 302 mg).

Table 18.5. Sodium Content of Processed Foods

CATEGORY	PRODUCT	AMOUNT	SODIUM (MG)
Breads	Pepperidge Farm White	2 slices	234
	Pepperidge Farm Whole Wheat	2 slices	355
Cereals	Kellogg's Corn Flakes	1 ounce	320
	Kellogg's Special K	1 ounce	227
	Kellogg's Sugar Frosted Flakes	1 ounce	186
Pancakes	Hungry Jack Extra Lights	3	1,150
Cheese	Breakstone's Lowfat Cottage Cheese	½ cup	435
	Kraft Processed American Cheese	1 ounce	238

Soups	Campbell's Tomato Soup	10 ounces	1,050
	Lipton Vegetable Cup-a-Soup	8 ounces	1,058
Beverages	Carnation Instant Hot Cocoa Mix	1 packet	104
Main courses	Morton King Size Turkey Dinner	1 dinner	2,567
	Swanson Fried Chicken Dinner	1 dinner	1,152
	Campbell's Beans and Franks	8 ounces	958
	Chef Boyardee Frozen Cheese Pizza	6 ounces	925
	Del Monte Tuna in oil	3 ounces	430
	Oscar Meyer Beef Franks	1 frank	425
Spreads	Skippy Peanut Butter	2 tbsp	167
Vegetables	B&M Brick Oven Baked Beans	1 cup	810
	Del Monte Whole Green Beans	1 cup	698
Fast foods	McDonald's Big Mac	1	962
	McDonald's Egg McMuffin	1	914
	Kentucky Fried Chicken	3 pieces	2,285
	McDonald's Apple Pie	1	414
	McDonald's Chocolate Shake	1	329
Snacks	Nabisco Premium Saltines	1 ounce	430
	Lay's Potato Chips	1 ounce	230
	Heinz Kosher Dill Pickle	1 large	1,137
Condiments	Wish-Bone Italian Dressing	1 tbsp	315
	Heinz Tomato Ketchup	1 tbsp	154
Desserts	Jell-O Chocolate Flavor Instant Pudding	½ cup	480
	Hostess Twinkies	1	190
	Pillsbury Cinnamon Raisin Danish	2 rolls	540
	Nabisco Oreo Cookies	3	240

Source: Adapted from *Jane Brody's Nutrition Book* (Toronto: Bantam, 1987).

BREAKING THE SALT HABIT

To have much effect on your blood pressure, you will probably need to cut your salt intake by at least 50 percent, or more if you're a salt guzzler. Knowing what foods to eat is only half the battle. The other half is actually getting used to low-salt foods, and sticking with them. The following are some of the tricks that people have found helpful.

- Avoid processed food whenever possible.
- Don't add salt to your food.
- Gradually reduce the amount of salt you use in cooking and baking. Start by using half the amount given in the recipe, and then reduce it further.
- Substitute herbs and spices for salt, to add flavor. Craig Claiborne, who has written many cookbooks, recommends onions, garlic, and pepper.

- Get yourself a low-salt cookbook.
- Avoid fast-food restaurants. Nearly all their foods are heavily salted as well as containing a lot of fat.

INCREASING YOUR POTASSIUM INTAKE

Potassium is found in a variety of foods including fruits, vegetables, meat, and milk. The recommended daily intake is about 2,000 milligrams. A serving of meat may contain up to 500 milligrams of potassium, so if you're cutting down on your meat intake you can make up the potassium by substituting one or more of the items shown in Table 18.6.

Table 18.6. Foods High in Potassium and Low in Sodium

FOOD	SERVING	POTASSIUM (mg)	SODIUM (mg)
Apricots	3 medium	281	1
Apricots (dried)	8 halves	490	13
Asparagus	6 spears	278	2
Avocado	1 half	604	4
Banana	1 medium	569	1
Beans (white)	½ cup	416	7
Beans (green)	1 cup	189	5
Broccoli	1 stalk	267	10
Cantaloupe	¼	251	12
Carrots	2 small	341	47
Dates	10	648	1
Grapefruit	½	135	1
Mushrooms	4 large	414	15
Orange	1 medium	311	2
Orange juice	1 cup	496	3
Peach	1 medium	202	1
Peanuts (plain)	2½ ounces	740	2
Potato	1 medium	504	4
Prunes (dried)	8 large	940	11
Raisins	¼ cup	271	10
Spinach	½ cup	291	45
Squash (acorn)	½ baked	749	2
Sunflower seeds	3½ ounces	920	30
Sweet potato	1 small	367	15
Tomato	1 small	244	3
Watermelon	1 slice	600	6

Source: *Health and Nutrition Newsletter,* Vol. 1, 1985.

GETTING ENOUGH CALCIUM

The recommended daily intake of calcium is about 1,000 milligrams. Postmenopausal women, who are at risk of osteoporosis, may need as much as 1,500 milligrams. The traditional way of getting calcium is by drinking milk, which doesn't need to include a lot of fat if you choose skim milk. The calcium content of various foods is shown in Table 18.7.

Table 18.7. Foods Rich in Calcium

CATEGORY	ITEM	SERVING SIZE	CALCIUM (MG)
Dairy	Whole milk	1 cup	288
	Skim milk	1 cup	296
	Yogurt	1 cup	272
	Swiss cheese	1 ounce	262
	Cheddar cheese	1 ounce	213
	American cheese	1 ounce	198
	Cottage cheese, creamed	½ cup	116
	Cottage cheese, dry curd	½ cup	90
Ice cream		½ cup	97
Fish	Sardines, with bones	3 ounces	372
	Salmon, canned, with bones	3 ounces	167
Shellfish	Oysters	¾ cup	170
Vegetables	Collard greens	½ cup	145
	Spinach, cooked	½ cup	106
	Mustard greens, cooked	½ cup	97
	Kale, cooked	½ cup	74
	Broccoli, cooked	½ cup	68
Fruit	Orange	1 medium	54
Corn muffin		1 medium	45

Source: Adapted from *Jane Brody's Nutrition Book* (Toronto: Bantam, 1987).

FISH, SHELLFISH, AND OMEGA-3 FATTY ACIDS

People who eat fish are at low risk of heart disease, as described in Chapter 4. Both fish and shellfish are low in saturated fat, and much of the fat that they do contain is in the form of omega-3 fatty acids, which are classed as "good fats" (see Chapter 4). The omega-3 content of various kinds of fish is shown in Table 18.8.

Table 18.8. Omega-3 Content of Seafood

SEAFOOD	TYPE	OMEGA-3 CONTENT (IN GRAMS PER 100 GRAMS OF FISH)
Fish	Mackerel	2.5
	Tuna	2.0
	Herring	1.7
	Salmon	1.0
	Anchovy	1.4
	Bluefish	1.2
	Striped bass	0.8
	Trout	0.6
	Halibut	0.5
	Grouper	0.3
	Cod	0.3
	Flounder	0.2
	Haddock	0.2
	Red snapper	0.2
	Swordfish	0.2
	Plaice	0.2
	Sole	0.1
Shellfish	Shrimp	0.5
	Mussel	0.5
	Soft-shell clam	0.4
	Scallops	0.2
	Lobster	0.2

Source: Adapted from *The Omega-3 Breakthrough,* by Julius Fast (Tucson: Body Press, 1987).

RECOMMENDED COOKBOOKS

The number of available diet books is almost limitless. The following list is not meant to be exhaustive, but includes books that focus on either the American Heart Association recommendations (low fat, low salt) or the Mediterranean diet. They all include information about the nutritional contents of the recipes (typically calories, fat, cholesterol, and sodium).

The Mediterranean Diet Cookbook. Nancy Harmon Jenkins. Bantam, 1994. $27.95.
   This is a wonderful book. It contains a rich variety of recipes from several

Mediterranean countries; it also discusses the Mediterranean diet and Food Pyramid.

Mediterranean Light. Delicious Recipes from the World's Healthiest Cuisine. Martha Rose Shulman. Bantam, 1989. $27.50.

This book also provides a large number of Mediterranean recipes, many of which have been modified to restrict the amount of fat and calories.

The American Heart Association Cookbook, 5th edition. Times Books, 1991. $14.00 (paperback).

The emphasis of this book, which contains 600 recipes, is on the Step One diet of the AHA. It has sold more than 1 million copies.

The American Heart Association Low-Fat, Low-Cholesterol Cookbook. Scott M. Grundy and Mary Winter, editors. Times Books, 1991. $13.00 (paperback).

This provides 200 recipes that are aimed at people with high cholesterol, and includes both the Step One and the Step Two diets.

Eat More, Weigh Less. Dean Ornish. Harper, 1994. $14.00 (paperback).

Dr. Ornish advocates an ultra-low-fat diet, in the form of 250 recipes such as tofu stew and bean burgers.

Brand Name Fat and Cholesterol Counter. American Heart Association. Times Books, 1994. $4.99.

This has no recipes, but gives the nutritional components of more than 4,000 brand-name foods.

The Sodium Counter. Annette B. Natow and Jo-Ann Heslin. Pocket Books, $4.99.

Written by the authors of *The Fat Counter* and *The Cholesterol Counter,* this gives the calorie and sodium content of 9,000 foods.

SUMMARY

• You can have only one type of diet: your objective should be a diet that minimizes your risk of cardiovascular disease and cancer, rather than simply lowering your blood pressure. Above all, it should be palatable.

• For most of us, restricting calories (which come mostly from fat) should be the top priority.

• The conventionally recommended low-fat diets such as the American Heart Association diets are not necessarily the best; I favor the Mediterranean diet, which restricts "land-mammal" saturated fat, and derives most of its fat from olive oil.

- Eat fish at least twice a week.

- The basis of a good diet is an emphasis on fruits, vegetables, and grains.

- Avoid processed foods as much as possible; they tend to be high in salt and fat.

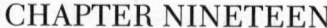

CHAPTER NINETEEN

LOSING WEIGHT

Without any doubt, weight loss is the most effective nondrug method of lowering blood pressure in people who are overweight. In theory it's also one of the easiest—you simply eat less; in practice, however, it's one of the hardest, as anyone who's tried to diet will tell you.

DIFFERING PERCEPTIONS OF BODY WEIGHT

In his novel *Bonfire of the Vanities,* Tom Wolfe gives a brilliant description of the fashionable notions of body weight in contemporary society. He describes the guests at a New York dinner party:

> The women came in two varieties. First, there were women in their late thirties and in their forties and older (women "of a certain age"), all of them skin and bones (starved to near perfection). To compensate for the concupiscence missing from their juiceless ribs and atrophied backsides, they turned to the dress designers. This season no puffs, flounces, pleats, ruffles, bibs, bows, battings, scallops, laces, darts, or shirrs on the bias were too extreme. They were the social X rays, to use the phrase that had bubbled up into Sherman's own brain. Second, there were the so-called lemon tarts. These were women in their twenties or early thirties, mostly blondes (the Lemon in the Tarts), who were the second, third, and fourth wives or live-in girlfriends of men over forty or fifty or sixty (or seventy), the sort of women men refer to, quite without thinking, as girls. This season the Tart was able to flaunt the natural advantages of youth by showing her legs from well above the knee and emphasizing her round bottom (something no X ray had). What was entirely missing from chez Bavardage was that manner of woman who is neither very young nor very old, who has laid in a lining of subcutaneous fat, who glows with plumpness and a rosy face that speaks,

without a word, of home and hearth and hot food ready at six and stories read aloud at night and conversations while seated on the edge of the bed, just before the sandman comes. In short, no one ever invited . . . Mother.

This "esthetic ideal" of what constitutes the desirable body weight is, of course, applied only to women, and explains why binge eating and bulimia are so much commoner in women than in men. It has nothing to do with health, and the "impeccably emaciated" women in Tom Wolfe's novel are probably less healthy than "Mother."

We'll next consider what is an ideal body weight from a health perspective.

WHAT IS MY IDEAL BODY WEIGHT?

Just as with blood pressure, there is no exact definition of whether someone is overweight or not. The traditional standards, which are shown in Table 19.1 for men, and in Table 19.2 for women, were derived by the Metropolitan Life Insurance Company. The acceptable weight range was taken as the one associated with the lowest mortality over a follow-up period of up to 30 years, and obesity as 20 percent above this range. People with large frames should be at the upper end of the range, and those with small frames at the lower end.

Table 19.1. Ideal Body Weights for Men

	WEIGHT WITHOUT CLOTHES (LB.)		
HEIGHT WITHOUT SHOES (FT., IN.)	ACCEPTABLE AVERAGE	ACCEPTABLE WEIGHT RANGE	OBESITY
5′ 2″	123	112–141	169
5′ 3″	127	115–144	173
5′ 4″	130	118–148	178
5′ 5″	133	121–152	182
5′ 6″	136	124–156	187
5′ 7″	140	128–161	193
5′ 8″	145	132–166	199
5′ 9″	149	136–170	204
5′ 10″	153	140–174	209
5′ 11″	158	144–179	215
6′ 0″	162	148–184	221
6′ 1″	166	152–189	227
6′ 2″	171	156–194	227
6′ 3″	176	160–199	239
6′ 4″	181	164–204	245

Table 19.2. Ideal Body Weights for Women

| HEIGHT WITHOUT SHOES (FT., IN.) | WEIGHT WITHOUT CLOTHES (LB.) | | |
	ACCEPTABLE AVERAGE	ACCEPTABLE WEIGHT RANGE	OBESITY
4′ 10″	102	92–119	143
4′ 11″	104	94–122	146
5′ 0″	107	96–125	150
5′ 1″	110	99–128	152
5′ 2″	113	102–131	154
5′ 3″	116	105–134	161
5′ 4″	120	108–138	166
5′ 5″	123	111–142	170
5′ 6″	128	114–146	175
5′ 7″	132	118–150	180
5′ 8″	136	122–154	185
5′ 9″	140	126–158	190
5′ 10″	144	130–163	196
5′ 11″	148	134–168	202
6′ 0″	152	138–173	208

WHY DIETS ARE DISAPPOINTING

Many people who go on a diet to lose weight are disappointed to find that very little happens, even though their intake of calories is greatly reduced. One reason for this is that our bodies can adapt to starvation by lowering the metabolic rate. While this ability may originally have been advantageous in evolutionary terms, by enabling people to survive longer during periods of starvation, it is today merely a source of frustration. It is also the reason why it's so important to combine dieting with exercise.

THE ANTIDIETING MOVEMENT

In reaction to the dieting craze in seeking the elusive esthetic ideal of the social X ray portrayed on the covers of women's magazines, feminist writers began a backlash movement against dieting. There were other reasons for this: the increasing recognition of serious eating disorders related to dieting, the frustration of women who had failed to lose weight when they dieted, and concerns about the adverse effects of the yo-yo weight cycle.

Their ranks have been joined by some of the leading obesity researchers. Dr. John Foreyt, of Baylor University in Houston, has said: "The worst thing a person can do about a weight problem is to go on a diet." His reasons for making this statement were that the body's metabolism slows down when faced with starvation, and that the dieter starts thinking and dreaming about food, suffers violent mood swings, and then turns to food as an emotional salve. He believes that the emphasis should be more on adopting a healthy lifestyle rather than becoming obsessed about dieting and weight.

SETTING YOURSELF A REASONABLE GOAL FOR LOSING WEIGHT

The television commercials and magazine advertisements for commercial weight-loss programs typically show before-and-after pictures of people who have magically lost 150 pounds. While such people presumably do exist, I have never met one. The tables of ideal weight shown above are a useful guide, and give the weight you should ultimately strive for; if you can do it, so much the better. But if you can't, don't despair; every pound that you lose and don't regain is a worthwhile achievement. Rather than saying you'll lose 25 pounds to get down to your ideal weight, and then getting frustrated when you don't, it's much better to start out by setting yourself an achievable goal of 10 pounds that you can maintain over the long term.

EAT MORE, WEIGH LESS—FACT OR FICTION?

You may recognize *Eat More, Weigh Less* as the title of Dr. Dean Ornish's latest book. It sounds too good to be true, and to a large extent it is. There is something to it, however. Dieting usually connotes eating less, but since different foods have very different caloric contents, it is in principle possible to lose weight by reducing the caloric content of one's food rather than by simply eating less. Thus there are studies that have shown that switching from a high-fat/low-carbohydrate diet to a low-fat/high-carbohydrate diet without altering the total amount of food eaten can result in weight loss.

The scientific basis for this finding is that carbohydrates have fewer calories than fats, and also that the more carbohydrate you eat, the more you burn. When you eat more fat, you don't burn it off, but simply store it as surplus energy.

This is the basis of Dr. Ornish's diet: you're allowed only 10 percent of the total calories as fat. This is a very tough call in practice: the average American diet contains 40 percent fat, and the generally recommended prudent diet is up to 30 percent. If you can stick with it, there is a good chance that it will work. A group of men who followed Dr. Ornish's program of diet and exercise lost 22 pounds on average, and managed to keep most of the weight off for up to 8 years.

There are in practice two major problems with this approach. The first is that if you are insulin-resistant (see Chapter 5 for a description of this), you won't burn up the extra carbohydrate, but store it as fat. The second is that there is a tendency for people to think that if they restrict fat they can eat as much as they like, which is quite wrong. A calorie is a calorie is a calorie. One of the commonest complaints heard by nutritionists these days is "How did I gain weight on a low-fat diet?" So beware those enticing "low-fat hot fudge sundaes." They *are* too good to be true.

STRATEGIES FOR SUCCESSFUL WEIGHT LOSS

For most people the idea of losing weight implies going on a diet, which means skipping meals, giving up the foods you like ("if it tastes good, don't eat it"), and generally making life miserable. While you may lose many pounds over the short term, the chances are overwhelming that you won't stick to it, and in a couple of months you'll be back where you started.

The secret of success is making gradual and small changes that you can live with over the long term. You will need to produce a small net calorie deficit, such that you burn more than you consume. Most people who have successfully lost weight say that the best way is a combination of decreased intake and increased expenditure by physical activity. A recent survey of the readers of *Prevention* magazine identified the following top 20 strategies.

1. Reducing fat intake.
2. Exercising regularly.
3. Reducing total calories.
4. Drinking more water.
5. Eating fewer sweets.
6. Keeping problem foods out of the house.
7. Walking for fitness.

8. Increasing high-fiber foods.
9. Reading food labels.
10. Keeping a food diary.
11. Eating low-fat foods.
12. Cutting back on meat intake.
13. Enjoying exercise.
14. Increasing self-esteem.
15. Planning what you'll eat.
16. Eating smaller but frequent meals.
17. Having a support group.
18. Doing aerobics.
19. Becoming more conscious of why you eat.
20. Reducing between-meal snacking.

You'll notice that there's a lot of overlap in this list: exercise appears four times (numbers 2, 7, 13, and 18) and reducing fat intake three times (1, 11, and 12). There are three general strategies here, which together give you a good chance of success.

Strategy One: Changing Your Eating Pattern

Decrease your fat intake. This is the number-one priority, and makes sense because fat contains twice as many calories as protein or carbohydrate, and if you focus on fat you'll probably cut down on carbohydrate intake as well, because the two often go together. One way you can do this is by eating less meat, which is one of the major sources of fat, particularly saturated fat. Another is by choosing low-fat substitutes for many of the foods you like: if you have a salad, choose an Italian dressing rather than blue cheese.

Eat high-fiber foods. Fiber is a very good way of filling your stomach, because it has a lot of bulk that takes a long time to digest. It also helps to lower your blood pressure and cholesterol.

Reduce portion size. If you're going to have steak, order a 4-ounce fillet rather than a 12-ounce T-bone.

Eat small but frequent meals. This helps to keep your blood sugar at a steady level, so you don't get excessively hungry. Skipping meals is not the way to lose weight. This does not mean that you should snack between meals.

Drink more water. When you're hungry, this is a good way of filling your stomach.

Strategy Two: Increasing Your Physical Activity

There are all sorts of ways that you can do this, which are discussed in Chapter 21.

Strategy Three: Taking Control of Your Life

There are several organizational things you can do that will make your task easier.

Think positive, getting the idea that you are in control of the situation, and that if you want to succeed you can.

Keep a food diary. This helps to get you into the habit of examining what you eat, and why. Hunger is often not the only reason for eating. Others include boredom, stress, and anger.

Plan what you're going to eat. If you plan your meals in advance rather than relying on impulsive decisions, you'll have a much better chance of choosing the right things.

Have a support group. There are many ways you can get support that will help to keep you going: your family, your friends, or an organized group (see below).

YO-YO DIETING—MORE HARM THAN GOOD?

There has been a lot of publicity about the adverse effects of yo-yo dieting, with alternating periods of weight loss and gain. At least three studies have shown that body weight fluctuation was associated with increased overall mortality, including from coronary heart disease, but not from cancer. No relationship was seen in two other studies. The largest such study was conducted by Dr. Ralph Paffenbarger, who followed the progress of nearly 12,000 middle-aged Harvard alumni over a 15-year period. When he looked at how their weight had changed during that time he found a U-shaped relationship between weight change and mortality: the lowest death rate from heart disease occurred in the men whose weight had remained the same, and higher rates were seen in men who had either gained or lost weight. The weight loss was not necessarily a gradual one, however. The men who weighed 10 pounds less after 15 years had in fact lost a total of 90 pounds over their lifetime, so they must also have put on 80 pounds. You might think that this means that if you are overweight you don't have to worry, but the same study showed that how overweight you are is much more important than how much your weight changes. Perhaps there are two lessons here: one is to try to avoid middle-aged spread—the insidious upward creep of body weight that happens to most of us, and the other is that if you are seriously overweight, crash diets are not the answer, since they almost always end up with yo-yo weight cycling.

COMMERCIAL WEIGHT-LOSS PROGRAMS

The American weight-loss industry is growing at a breathtaking rate. Ten billion dollars were spent on it in 1989, and it has been estimated that this will be $50 billion soon. The programs that have claimed most attention are the proprietary "very-low-calorie diet" programs, of which Optifast, promoted by the Sandoz pharmaceutical company, is the best known. Extravagant claims have been made for these programs, which have hitherto been subjected to little governmental regulation. However, the Federal Trade Commission (FTC) has now initiated an intensive review of these programs.

There are two basic types of commercial weight-loss programs. The first utilizes low-calorie foods (800–1,200 calories per day), and the second is the more drastic liquid diets (800 calories or less).

LOW-CALORIE DIET PROGRAMS—WEIGHT WATCHERS, NUTRI/SYSTEM, JENNY CRAIG, AND DIET CENTER

These programs typically recommend specific meal programs with restricted calories. The food required can usually be purchased at the supermarket, but some programs require that the specific food items be purchased at their clinics. These may consist of powdered supplements to be mixed with milk, dehydrated prepackaged food entrees, frozen food entrees, and snack bars. Participants in the programs visit the clinic weekly. They are designed to produce a weight loss of about 1 percent per week and to provide about 1,000 to 1,200 calories per day.

These programs usually offer advice on behavior modification, either individually or in groups. The instructors include successful past dieters, dietitians, and behavioral counselors. Physicians are not normally involved. None of the commercial programs has published their success rates in the medical literature.

Weight Watchers. This company, which is owned by H. J. Heinz, is the leader in the industry, with $300 million in sales annually and 5 million members. The program uses a list of regular foods that can be purchased at any grocery, which keeps the costs low. You also pay for weekly meetings, with public weighing of all the group members and instruction in behavior modification and exercise. The diets are well balanced and, since they involve no special foods, can be followed indefinitely.

Nutri/System. Prepackaged food entrees are purchased at the clinic, and fruits and vegetables are bought at a grocer's. The cost of the program is determined by the weight loss required to achieve your ideal body weight.

Jenny Craig. This program is similar to Nutri/System, except that it charges a flat rate regardless of the amount of weight that needs to be lost. Ninety-five percent of its members are women, for whom part of its appeal is the prepackaged food ("Jenny's Cuisine"), which obviates the need for food preparation.

Diet Center. Food purchases are made outside the clinic, but dairy products are eliminated, and replaced by a soy protein supplement purchased in the clinic. The fees are determined by the required weight loss.

MEDICALLY SUPERVISED LIQUID PROTEIN DIETS— OPTIFAST, MEDIFAST, AND HMR

Because they employ a much more drastic restriction of calories, the liquid diet programs require close medical supervision. They are recommended only for people who are more than 30 percent overweight. Calories are restricted to fewer than 800 per day. They consist mainly of protein in order to prevent loss of muscle tissue. Their purpose is to promote a weight loss of about 2 percent per week for a period of 12 weeks.

Like any other form of medical treatment, they can have side effects. These include fatigue, hair loss, and dizziness, all of which are transient. The most serious one is an increased risk of gallstones.

The effectiveness of such programs was recently reviewed in a study conducted by two of the leading experts in the field of obesity, Drs. Thomas Wadden and Albert Stunkard. They followed the progress of 517 men and women who completed a six-month Optifast program. This included 12 weeks of a liquid diet, with 800 calories per day, followed by a gradual transition to a regular low-calorie diet. The participants were enrolled in groups, and received counseling from a behavioral counselor, a dietitian, and an exercise physiologist.

The results can be summarized as follows:

- Just over half of the participants completed the program.
- Women lost 21 percent of their body weight, and men 25 percent.
- In those participants who were hypertensive (about 10 percent of the total) the blood pressure fell from 147/93 mm Hg to 125/80.
- Blood cholesterol fell from 218 to 187 mg/dl.
- One year after completing the study, just over a third of the weight lost had been regained, although about 20 percent of the participants succeeded in maintaining the full amount of weight lost.

The authors commented that one reason for the relatively good results was the group sessions, an important feature of which was that the membership of the groups was the same throughout the study.

OVER-THE-COUNTER LIQUID DIETS—SLIMFAST, DYNATRIM

These are meal replacement drinks that usually replace two meals; the third is intended to be a calorie-controlled meal. Each drink contains 200 calories. They are easy to use, because no meal preparation is involved, but there is also no flexibility, and there is no incentive to develop new and more healthy eating patterns. Like most of the other commercial programs, there are no published results.

SUPPORT GROUPS

Everyone has heard of Alcoholics Anonymous, the group of former alcoholics who provide moral support for people who are trying to kick the habit. Similar groups have been organized to help the overweight in their struggle to be thin. Two of the best known are Overeaters Anonymous (OA) and Take Off Pounds Sensibly (TOPS). They do not provide specific dietary advice, but give support and motivation.

RECOMMENDED DIET BOOKS

For many of the major publishing companies, diet books are their bread and butter. The public's appetite for them seems to be as strong as their appetite for ice cream. Unfortunately, there's more to losing weight than buying the latest book about it. Frances Berg, editor of *Obesity and Health Newsletter*, advises caution: "Don't waste your time with books that use terms like 'miraculous,' 'breakthrough,' 'exclusive,' 'secret,' 'ancient,' 'unique,' or 'accidental discovery.' And if it claims or implies quick, easy weight loss, look the other way."

The best are ones written by professional nutritionists; some of the worst are written by physicians. Here is a list that was recommended by Densie Webb in *The New York Times*.

The Choose to Lose Diet, by Dr. Ron Goor, Nancy Goor, and Katherine Boyd. Houghton Mifflin, 1990.

Everywoman's Guide to Nutrition, by Judith Brown. University of Minnesota Press, 1991.

The Duke University Medical Center Book of Diet and Fitness. Fawcett Columbine, 1991.

The Tufts University Guide to Total Nutrition, by Stanley Gershoff. Harper-Collins, 1991.

Eating Smart: ABC's of The New Food Literacy, by Jeanne Jones. Macmillan, 1992.

The New American Diet System, by Sonja L. and William E. Connor. Simon & Schuster, 1991.

Controlling Your Fat Tooth, by Joseph C. Piscatella. Workman, 1991.

DIET PILLS

If obesity is a chronic condition that, like diabetes and hypertension, leads to serious complications, why not also treat it with medications? The idea certainly makes sense, and is slowly gaining acceptance in medical circles, but it's an uphill struggle. Appetite suppressants have been around for a long time, but got themselves a bad name because the original ones were derived from amphetamine, which is an addictive drug. In the past few years interest in them has been renewed as the result of a four-year study conducted at the University of Rochester and funded by the National Institutes of Health (NIH) using two newer drugs, fenfluramine hydrochloride and phentermine hydrochloride, which are relatively free of adverse effects. Obese subjects were given the usual advice about diet and exercise, and allocated to take either the two appetite suppressants (phentermine and fenfluramine) or placebo (dummy) pills. The reason for giving the two drugs in combination was that one of them (phentermine, which is related to amphetamine) is a mild stimulant, whereas the other (fenfluramine, which works differently) is a sedative. In combination, these two effects cancel each other out. The subjects taking the medications lost more weight than the others, but when they stopped taking them at the end of the study, nearly four years later, their weight slowly rose again. The main side effect was a dry mouth (which became less noticeable with time), and there was no evidence of abuse or addiction.

Neither of the drugs is new, although this was the first study to examine their combined use over a long period. Fenfluramine is sold under the brand name Pondimin, and phentermine as Ionamin, Adipex-P, Fastin, and Phentermine HCl. Despite the encouraging results of the NIH study, both are classified by the FDA as addictive drugs, which means that they are not supposed to be taken for more than 12 weeks at a time.

It seems to me that if you have a chronic weight problem that has not responded to diet and exercise, you should give serious consideration to trying these drugs, and that the FDA viewpoint is unnecessarily alarmist. Discuss it with your doctor.

THE COST OF LOSING

It is unfortunate that one individual's excess weight should be another's source of income, but the weight-loss industry is as competitive and aggressive as any other. If you decide that a commercial weight-loss program is for you, you're certainly going to want to know how much the different programs cost. A recent survey revealed that there are in fact huge differences between the costs of different programs. The most expensive of the low-calorie food programs (Jenny Craig) might cost $1,025 for 12 weeks, while the cheapest (Weight Watchers) would cost only $108. However, when comparing such costs you should remember that the cost of a program such as Jenny Craig includes all the costs of food except for fresh fruits and vegetables and drinks. The liquid diet programs are more expensive, ranging from $2,120 (United Weight Control) to $1,140 (Medifast) for the same amount of weight lost. In these programs the only additional costs are for low-calorie drinks. The extra expense of these programs is largely due to the intense medical supervision required.

SUMMARY

• Set yourself a reasonable goal for losing weight; if you can achieve and maintain a 10-pound loss, you've done well.

• Crash or fad diets are not the answer.

• Fat has twice as many calories as carbohydrate or protein, so switch from fatty and processed foods to fruit and vegetables.

• Cut down on portion sizes; if you need to fill up, eat high-fiber food.

• Increase your level of physical activity.

CHAPTER TWENTY

QUITTING SMOKING

If you have high blood pressure and you smoke, you're at much greater risk of getting a heart attack or a stroke than if you have either risk factor on its own, as we saw in Chapter 7. And of the two, smoking is much the more important: you can cut your risk five times more by quitting smoking than by having your pressure lowered. So that's good news. The other piece of good news is that people are quitting in large numbers. In 1965 about 40 percent of the American population smoked; today that number is down to about a quarter. Smoking is no longer viewed as sophisticated behavior; the model for the Marlboro Man, looking cool under his Stetson, in reality died of lung cancer. The groups that have been most resistant to this trend are blacks and the poor—ironically, the people who can least afford the cost of smoking and its consequences.

SMOKING IS AN ADDICTION

Smoking has been formally recognized as an addiction by the World Health Organization and the Surgeon General. This comes as no surprise to smokers, 70 percent of whom recognize that they are addicted without being told. The addiction takes three forms—chemical, psychological, and social. That, of course, is why it's so hard to kick the habit. The ingredient of tobacco smoke that is responsible for the chemical addiction is nicotine, which is also the ingredient that makes smoking enjoyable in the first place. In low doses, nicotine produces a feeling of alertness; some people say that they need a cigarette to get them started in the morning, others that it helps them concentrate while at work. At higher doses, it can have a calming effect, as in the example of the condemned man who requests one last cigarette before he goes to his execution. And it works within a few seconds of inhaling, which is another reason why it's so addictive. So the experienced smoker can get the desired effect by varying the rate of puffing. Like other addictive drugs (heroin, alcohol, and cocaine) long-term use results in the development of tolerance, so that withdrawal symptoms occur during periods of abstinence. As few as two cigarettes may be enough to get someone hooked: about half of adolescents who smoke two or more cigarettes become habitual smokers. Also in common with other addictive drugs is a very high relapse rate in people who try to quit—about 70 percent are smoking again after three months.

The trouble with giving up smoking, like any other form of chemical addiction, is that you smoke not just for the pleasure it brings, but much more to avoid the pain of withdrawal when you don't. This is the theory behind the use of nicotine chewing gum and patches, which help to some extent but give no magic cures. That's because there's also a psychological component to the addiction—the rituals of lighting up, holding the cigarette in your fingers, the Freudian act of sucking on it, and so on.

The third barrier to overcome is a social one, which is the pressure exerted by your peers. This is one of the main reasons why teenagers start; they think it's cool, as the advertisements for Camels have emphasized so effectively. Fortunately, this is one barrier that's steadily being dismantled, as the social pressures against smoking increase.

CAN I SWITCH TO LOW-NICOTINE CIGARETTES OR CIGARS?

You guessed it—the answer to this question is no. In principle, low-nicotine cigarettes are less damaging than Lucky Strikes, but what will happen is that you'll simply inhale more, to get the same nicotine high as before. Studies have been done of the blood levels of nicotine in smokers, which have shown no difference between those smoking light cigarettes and those who smoke the full-flavored sort. Also, if you've been a cigarette smoker all your life and you switch to a pipe or cigars, the chances are that you'll inhale the smoke for the same reason. So you're back to square one. Smoking pipes and cigars carries additional risks such as cancer of the mouth and esophagus.

Switching to chewing tobacco is also not an answer: you still get the nicotine damaging your arteries, and it also causes cancer of the mouth, as well as gum disease.

How to Quit Smoking

The first thing to state is that there is no magic formula; the second is that anyone can quit if he or she really wants to. Most people who smoke say they would like to quit but, for one reason or another, can't. Giving up any form of addiction is not easy. Every year about 17 million smokers in the United States try to quit, but fewer than one in ten are successful. Most people don't succeed on their first attempt, but if they keep trying, the chances improve. And 37 million Americans have eventually made it, mostly on their own. You could be one of them.

Before you actually quit, it's a good idea to do some planning. Choose a day in advance, and then tell your spouse, your friends, and the people you work with, so that they can give you moral support when the time comes, and if they smoke, they can avoid doing so in your presence. Make a list of the times and situations when you normally like to smoke, and think about how you might deal with them. If, for example, you smoke after a meal, plan some other activity, and when you've finished eating, get up right away and start doing it. Or if you smoke while watching television, you might get in a supply of carrot or celery sticks to nibble on instead of having a cigarette. Another helpful trick is to learn to take regular deep breaths and make an effort to relax when you get the urge to light up. You might also plan to arrange your calendar so that you avoid situations where you'd be most likely to smoke; instead of going out with friends who smoke, for example, you might plan to go to a movie.

You should also start to think about the positive aspects of quitting: your food will taste better, you'll breathe more easily, and you won't need an ashtray. Make a list of things on which you might spend the money you'll save by not smoking.

A Seven-Day Program for Quitting Smoking

This program was recommended to the employees of New York Hospital when it became a smoke-free environment.

Day 1

- List all your reasons for quitting. Review them daily.
- Throw away all your cigarettes, and then buy a brand you don't like.
- Don't empty ashtrays.

Day 2

- Review your quit list.
- Before smoking a cigarette, think about it for 10 seconds.
- Substitute celery, carrots, or sugarless gum for cigarettes.

Day 3

- Set a time during the day not to smoke (two hours for heavy smokers, half a day for light smokers).
- Try a deep breathing exercise instead of smoking: relax, and breathe in and out deeply three or four times.

Day 4

- Smoke only when you feel desperate for a cigarette.
- Treat yourself to a special dinner.
- Throw away your matches and lighters.

Day 5

- Buy no more cigarettes: smoke only when in dire need.
- Tell your friends that you are quitting; get encouragement.
- At the end of the day, wash ashtrays and hide them in a cabinet.

Day 6

- Don't smoke today.
- Make plans to visit museums, movies, or nonsmoking friends—places where smoking is prohibited!
- Avoid alcohol, which stimulates the urge to smoke.

Day 7

- Don't smoke today.
- Open a savings account for the money you save on cigarettes.
- Review your list of reasons to quit smoking; keep low-calorie snacks on hand and remember breathing exercises.
- If you have a cigarette, don't be discouraged. Start again on the QUIT SMOKING DAY you think is right. You can do it!

SMOKING CESSATION GROUPS AND CLINICS

If you've tried to quit on your own, and haven't succeeded, you may want to think about getting professional help. Fortunately, there are a lot of options. There are two general categories of programs. The first is those organized by nonprofit organizations, such as the Seventh-Day Adventists' Five-Day Plan, the American Lung Association's Freedom From Smoking clinics, and the American Cancer Society's FreshStart program. They all require a considerable investment of time and money; the American Lung Association's program may be the most effective, but it also requires a greater time commitment than the others.

The second category is the commercial programs, such as Smok-Enders, Smoke Stoppers, Smokeless, and Schick. Not surprisingly, they are substantially more expensive than the nonprofit programs, and they're not necessarily any more effective.

OTHER WAYS OF HELPING YOU QUIT, INCLUDING NICOTINE REPLACEMENT THERAPY

Going cold turkey, as in the program outlined above or in many of the clinic programs, is not for everyone and doesn't always work. There are several other possibilities that may help you achieve your goal. It's important to realize that none of them are substitutes for willpower—unless you have consciously decided that you really do want to quit, they're all a waste of time. We'll review some of them now.

The most effective methods are the nicotine replacement therapies, in which the nicotine you normally get from cigarettes is replaced by nicotine in another form, which is designed to separate the chemical addiction from the behavioral dependency on smoking. These come in various forms: the original one was nicotine gum, but this has largely been replaced by patches, nasal sprays, and inhalers.

Nicotine Chewing Gum

Because of the chemical addiction associated with nicotine, a form of nicotine substitution therapy has been developed, similar to methadone substitution for heroin addicts. Chewing gum is impregnated with nicotine, which is gradually absorbed through the mouth into the circulation. It's available only on prescription, but has become very popular: over $100 million worth was sold in 1990. The gum serves two purposes: first, to prevent nicotine withdrawal symptoms at the time of quitting smoking, and second, to provide a substitute oral activity. The recommended way of using the gum is to practice chewing it for a few days before the target quitting day, and on the target day to quit smoking abruptly. The gum is then chewed whenever the urge to smoke gets very strong. Its use is continued for four months, after which it is gradually reduced. It works well only if these guidelines are followed:

- Tobacco is completely avoided while using the gum.
- The gum is used as part of a structured smoking cessation program.
- Ten to 12 pieces of gum are used per day for one to three months.

In practice, this is often not the way the gum is used. In many cases the patient asks the doctor for a prescription, and then does not follow the recommended procedure; many use it for less than a month, which is usually too short a time for it to be really effective. Even worse, some people use it in situations where smoking is not allowed, so they may actually be increasing their nicotine dependency.

Very few smokers enjoy chewing the gum at first, though some get to like it later. If it is chewed too fast it can cause excessive salivation and irritation of the tongue. It's been found to be moderately successful in some studies, but is no panacea. It's most helpful in the early stages of quitting.

Nicotine Skin Patches

The recent approval by the FDA of nicotine patches, which go by the names of Nicoderm, Habitrol, and Prostep, has been a real bonanza for the pharmaceutical corporations, which have even advertised them on prime-time television. The theory underlying their use is that they release a steady supply of nicotine into the bloodstream (to reach a level about 50 percent of what is obtained by smoking one and a half packs per day), so that the psychological component of smoking can be divorced from the chemical component of the addiction, and by gradually tapering the dose of nicotine over a period of several weeks, the agony of withdrawal symptoms can be avoided.

The patches come in three strengths, and the idea is to use one patch per day of each strength for about a month, starting with the strongest and tapering down to the weakest. The cost is about $30 per week.

There have been at least 10 well-controlled clinical trials of the nicotine patches, in each of which they were compared with (inert) placebo patches. Most of the trials provided little or no professional counseling, so that they simulated the way in which the patches are most commonly used. Nine out of 10 trials found that the patches worked better than the placebo (measured by the number of people who actually succeeded in quitting). Nicotine patches are also more effective than nicotine gum.

Just as with the nicotine gum, it's crucial that the patches be used as part of a structured smoking cessation program. The first one goes on during the morning of "quit day." The main side effect of the patches is skin irritation.

How Effective Are Nicotine Replacement Therapies?

There have been a number of controlled clinical trials of the effectiveness of this new form of treatment, in which one group of smokers who were prescribed the nicotine replacement therapy were compared with a control group who were merely given advice. A recent analysis by Professor Christopher Silagy and his colleagues looked at the results of 53 such trials, of which 42 used the gum, 9 the patch, 1 the spray, and 1 the inhaler. The total number of smokers taking part in these trials was nearly 18,000. The results are shown in Table 20.1.

Table 20.1. The Chances of Quitting Smoking Using Nicotine Replacement Therapy In Comparison with Advice Only

THERAPY	IMPROVEMENT IN CHANCE OF QUITTING
Inhaler	3.0 times
Nasal spray	2.9 times
Patch	2.1 times
Gum	1.6 times

All four forms of treatment produced significant improvements in the chances of quitting by the end of one year, but the best appeared to be the inhaler, where there was a threefold improvement, and the gum the least good. Like any other form of smoking cessation treatment, however, the relapse rate was high after the trials were completed, unless there was also intensive follow-up treatment.

OTHER PRODUCTS FOR SMOKING CESSATION

None of the products listed below is judged to be effective, but I will list them so you don't waste money on them.

Nikoban, Bantron. These contain a substance called lobeline, which is related to nicotine.

Healthbreak. This contains silver acetate, which produces an unpleasant taste in your mouth when you smoke a cigarette.

Cigarrest. This contains lobeline and some other substances.

Nicotine Filters. An example of these is called One Step At A Time. The filters are supposed to extract most of the nicotine, but what may happen is that you puff more frequently, or inhale more deeply. There's no evidence that they produce any long-term benefit.

Lifesign. This is a small hand-held computer that you can program so that it tells you when to smoke. Again, there are no data to show that it works.

HYPNOSIS

Virtually every city in the United States has a professional hypnotist, and smokers are their bread and butter. A typical session would be as follows. The therapist seats you in a comfortable chair and asks you to close your eyes and then to imagine that your arm is very light and floating up. He then repeats a series of messages, such as "Cigarettes are a poison for your body" or "You owe your body respect and protection." You are then instructed in self-hypnosis, and told to use it whenever you get the urge to smoke.

Although extravagant claims have been made for the cure rate with hypnosis, there have been few if any well-controlled studies, so I would be skeptical about it.

ACUPUNCTURE

Although acupuncture can produce some impressive anesthetic effects, claims that it can help you quit smoking are poorly substantiated.

AVERSION TECHNIQUES

Several commercial programs, such as Smoke Stoppers, Schick, and Smoking Cessation Centers, have incorporated aversion procedures.

The most commonly used have been rapid smoking and oversmoking, which are designed to increase your dislike for smoking, because an excess of nicotine may make you nauseated and even induce vomiting. While their effectiveness has been documented, they're not without risks, one of which is that they may increase your nicotine dependency.

WHAT IF YOU RELAPSE?

As many as 80 percent of smokers who initially succeed at stopping smoking will go back to it within a year. More than half require three or more attempts before they finally succeed. As Mark Twain said: "To cease smoking is the easiest thing I ever did; I ought to know because I've done it a thousand times." A recent report by the National Heart, Lung, and Blood Institute concluded: "We know how to help people quit smoking, and we are rather successful at it; we know little about how to prevent relapse, and we fail miserably." Smoking one cigarette after you've quit doesn't necessarily mean that you're doomed to going back to your old habits, although, of course, all relapses start with that one cigarette. You should be on your guard against situations that are known to be risk factors for relapses. One of the most important ones is stress: if one of the reasons you smoked in the first place was to cope with stress, when things get tough at work or at home you will surely be tempted to relapse. Another potentially dangerous time is when you're enjoying a few drinks with friends who smoke, and one of them offers you a cigarette. My wife quit successfully nearly twenty years ago, and this is the one situation in which she would now ever smoke.

When you first quit smoking, you should not assume that it's not going to last, but if you do relapse, don't despair. You may have lost the battle, but you can still win the war. It's up to you.

SUMMARY

- If you smoke, quitting is, quite literally, a matter of life and death.

- There's no magic formula for quitting; the first step is to convince yourself that you really want to.

- Plan your quitting program in advance, and try to get the support of friends and relatives.

- Nicotine patches can improve your chances of success.

- If at first you don't succeed, try again!

CHAPTER TWENTY-ONE

STARTING TO EXERCISE

A regular exercise program is good in all sorts of ways, not only for help-ing to control your blood pressure. In fact, even if it has no discernible effect on your pressure, I would still recommend it. I discussed some of the benefits in Chapter 6, but I will summarize them here.

THE BENEFITS OF REGULAR EXERCISE

- Your blood pressure will probably be lower. On average, you can expect your pressure to be up to 5 mm Hg lower if you exercise regularly, but this doesn't always happen.
- Your risk of heart disease will be lower. This was also discussed in Chapter 6.
- Your risk of having a stroke will also be reduced.
- Your HDL cholesterol will be higher. This means that you are less likely to lay down atherosclerotic plaques in your arteries.
- It will help keep your weight down. Exercise is an integral part of any good weight-loss program, and as well as burning calories, it helps preserve muscle mass. It will also help you keep your weight stable when you're trying to give up smoking.
- It helps control diabetes. The type of diabetes that is particularly associated with high blood pressure is due to insulin resistance, which exercise helps to overcome.
- It helps prevent osteoporosis. Like muscles, bones tend to get weak if they're not used, in this case for bearing weight (loss of bone is a major problem with long space flights). So a regular exercise pro-gram, which includes some weight lifting, helps keep them strong and prevent osteoporosis.

- It's good for your psyche. Not only will you look better without your beer belly, but you'll feel better. My wife, who is very healthy, hates exercise, but does it simply because she feels better all day if she's exercised in the morning. There is also evidence that it may help to prevent or treat depression.
- It helps you cope with aging. Physical disability in old people is a major problem, and in part it's a vicious cycle. As you get older you become less active, perhaps because you have some arthritis, so your bones and muscles get weaker, so you can do less, and so on. I take the view that you're never too old to exercise, and in fact some of the most dramatic results with exercise programs have been obtained in octogenarians (see Chapter 6).

SOME COMMON EXCUSES FOR NOT EXERCISING

I hate exercising. The usual reason for this is that people find it boring, so after they've done it a few times, they quit. The trick is to find a form of exercise that you like and can stick with, or to vary what you do from day to day. The choices are almost infinite, and many of them are discussed in the following pages. Another thing that you can do is to have something to occupy your mind while you exercise. Lots of people wear a Walkman while they exercise, and you can even get specially recorded tapes of music that have the right rhythm for what you are doing. If you have a stationary bicycle, you can put a television set in front of it, so you can watch the news while you pedal.

I don't have the time. Actually, the amount of time that you need to get the benefits from exercise is not very much—about 30 minutes three times a week should do. Just think about how much time you spend watching television, and also consider the possibility that you could be exercising at the same time. Furthermore, you'll get the time back in terms of increased productivity.

I'm too tired to exercise. This is in fact a good reason to start exercising! If you exercise you will have more mental and physical energy than if you don't.

I'm too old to exercise. You're never too old to do some form of exercise; you may not be able to ride a bike, but you could still lift weights or walk.

Exercise may be dangerous. I go into this question in more detail below; in general, however, the dangers of not exercising are greater than the dangers associated with exercise.

I'm afraid of getting injured. There's no doubt that exercise can cause injuries, and when it happens to a professional athlete such as a football player it gets a lot of publicity. Long-distance runners may get stress fractures, but for the average person such as you and me this should not be an issue. Activities such as walking, swimming, and bicycling cause virtually no increased strain on your joints. The only potential problem is that if you do too much too soon you may strain a muscle, but it will heal rapidly.

CAN EXERCISE BE DANGEROUS?

A common concern of people with high blood pressure is the risk of something bad happening while they're exercising. If your pressure is high to begin with, and goes even higher during exercise, isn't there a risk of bursting a blood vessel? This is a perfectly reasonable concern, but happily is not borne out by the evidence. People do drop dead while they're exercising, of course, and when it happens, it often gets reported on the news. A famous example was Jim Fixx, who wrote the best-selling book *The Complete Book of Running* and died while on a training run. Several studies have examined the factors that make people susceptible to this. Two conditions account for the majority of cases, and hypertension is not one of them. In young people, the commonest cause is a heart disorder called hypertrophic cardiomyopathy, which is characterized by an overgrowth of the heart muscle. Blood pressure is normal in these individuals. In people of middle age, the commonest predisposing cause is coronary heart disease. Jim Fixx had been experiencing chest pains before he died and had refused the offer of a stress test. Even in people who do have coronary heart disease, however, most experts would agree that the benefits of a regular exercise program outweigh the risks.

It is generally true that heart attacks are more likely to happen when people are active than when they are resting—they are relatively uncommon during sleep, for example. But most of the heart attacks that occur during exercise are in people who do not exercise regularly. That's another reason why we recommend that when you start to exercise you build up gradually and that you do it regularly. That way, you'll stay out of trouble.

Another fear that can be allayed is the risk of having a stroke from a burst blood vessel in the brain, or cerebral hemorrhage. In a study of 225 cases of cerebral hemorrhage leading to sudden death, most of which occurred in people who had high blood pressure, there was no association between the onset of symptoms and strenuous physical activity. The most common concurrent activity was walking, followed by working. There is thus no evidence that recreational exercise puts hypertensive individuals at any increased risk.

ARE THERE TIMES WHEN I SHOULDN'T EXERCISE?

It's not a good idea to exercise when you have any sort of infection, whether it be a cold or the flu.

SHOULD I HAVE A STRESS TEST BEFORE STARTING TO EXERCISE?

A number of health clubs ask for this before you can sign on, but it's largely done for medicolegal purposes. If you're basically healthy, and have no history of heart problems, it's probably not necessary, and may even be misleading, since a stress test may indicate that you have a problem when you really don't (this is particularly true in people with high blood pressure). Technically, this is known as a false-positive test, and occurs because there may be reasons other than coronary heart disease that cause the electrocardiogram (on which the results are based) to change during exercise. Furthermore, the stress test may not show any abnormality when in fact you do have heart disease (a false-negative result).

Knowing how high your pressure goes while you exercise is of limited value in practice, because a marked increase in systolic pressure is perfectly normal, and also because when you do your exercise program you may be doing a different type of exercise, and at a lower level, than during a stress test.

WHAT TYPE OF EXERCISE IS BEST?

Most of the studies that have shown the benefits of exercise in lowering blood pressure have used either running or bicycling, but any type of aerobic or dynamic exercise is likely to be equally beneficial. The best conditioning effects are obtained by exercising large muscle groups, which in practice means your legs. If you choose a relatively light form of exercise you'll need to do more of it to get the full benefits than if you do heavy exercise. As a general rule of thumb, burning 1,500 to 2,000 calories per week is about right. Table 21.1 shows how many calories you burn with different types of exercise.

Table 21.1. Calorie Expenditure with Different Types of Exercise

Activity	Calories Expended per Hour
Walking (2 mph)	240
Bicycling (6 mph)	240
Swimming (25 yd/min)	275
Walking (3 mph)	320
Tennis (singles)	400
Bicycling (12 mph)	410
Walking (4.5 mph)	440
Swimming (50 yd/min)	500
Running (5.5 mph)	740
Jumping rope	750
Running (7 mph)	920

Many people resent the idea of having to set aside a special part of the day to exercise, particularly if this means having to change clothes and go to a gym, but to get most of the benefits, there is an alternative solution, which was recently advocated by a joint recommendation from the federal Centers for Disease Control and the American College of Sports Medicine. This was that repeated light bouts of activity may produce nearly as much benefit as a sustained period of heavy exercise. Examples given were climbing stairs instead of using the elevator, and walking part of the way home instead of taking the bus all the way.

WALKING

Here's one form of exercise that anyone can do, and if you do enough of it, it's all you need. You can do it anywhere, anytime, and the only equipment you need is a pair of comfortable shoes. It can, of course, be a social activity as well as a physical one, and if you do it regularly with your spouse or a friend, you're more likely to stick with it. The main problem is the weather; one way around this that is becoming increasingly popular is to walk in a shopping mall, where there may even be mall-walking clubs. You don't need to walk particularly fast (although you'll burn more calories if you do)—3 or 4 miles an hour is fine.

RUNNING

This is one of my favorites, and has the advantage of being something that you can do almost anywhere and any time. The only equipment you need is a pair of shoes. It's also a good way of burning a lot of calories in a relatively short time. The President's Council on Physical Fitness and Sports rated running the number-one type of exercise.

Like any other form of exercise, you should not try to do too much at first. The experts recommend a warm-up period of stretching before you start.

BICYCLING

Almost all of us learned how to ride a bicycle when we were young, but you may not have been on one for many years. You can do it on a stationary bike in your own home, or you can venture forth on the road. The recent popularity of mountain bikes has revolutionized the sport, and means that you can go just about anywhere. One of the advantages over walking is that you can go much farther from home in the same time.

Bicycling normally exercises your legs, but not your arms. You still get the cardiovascular conditioning effect, of course, but if you want to get your arms into shape as well, there are stationary bikes that you can pedal with your arms as well as your legs.

CROSS-COUNTRY SKIING MACHINES

Cross-country skiing machines, such as NordicTrack, which simulate the activity of cross-country skiing, have become very popular, for one good reason: they provide a workout for your arms as well as your legs.

SWIMMING AND AQUA-AEROBICS

One of the advantages of swimming is that you put absolutely no pressure on your joints, so if you have back problems or arthritis, it's ideal. It also conditions your arms as well as your legs, which is another advantage. Its main limitation is the availability of a pool: unless you're lucky enough to have your own you're likely to have to travel some distance to get to one.

It does not matter what stroke you use; choose whichever one you feel most comfortable with.

Another type of exercise to be performed in a swimming pool is aqua-aerobics, which is advocated by Dr. Kenneth Cooper in his book *Overcoming Hypertension*. These are exercises that you can do while standing in the pool or holding on to its side. You get your exercise by moving the different parts of your body through the resistance of the water.

A further refinement on this theme is to get yourself a "Wet Vest"; this gives you enough buoyancy to float in the water, so that you can "walk" or "run" in deep water without sinking. It's ideal for small pools.

TENNIS

Here's another form of exercise that occupies your mind as well as your body. It's not for everyone, of course, and requires the availability of both a court and a partner of about your standard of play. You use more calories with singles than doubles; theoretically it's not as good for the cardiovascular system as some of the other forms of exercise because the exercise is not performed at a steady level. If you play, it's a good idea to combine it with another type of exercise.

The same things apply to other ball games such as squash and racquetball.

WEIGHT LIFTING (FREE WEIGHTS)

One activity that can really put your blood pressure through the roof is lifting heavy weights, such as barbells and dumbbells. Those burly men that you see on television during the Olympic weight-lifting competition with popping eyes and a big leather belt to stop their stomach from popping too may have a systolic pressure between 300 and 400 mm Hg. So don't do it.

Nautilus Machines

Weight lifting is a far cry from the modern resistance training or Nautilus machines. The key here is not to lift the maximum amount of weight, but to lift a smaller load several times in quick succession. This doesn't make the blood pressure go up so much, and is better for strength training as well as conditioning. The machines let you choose how much weight you will lift, and you should choose a level at which you can do 10 or 15 repetitions within 45 seconds. By using the different machines that are available at most health clubs, you can exercise just about every muscle in your body. You can also get home versions, some of which are reasonably priced and enable you to do a number of different exercises on the same machine.

Dancing

This has to be one sort of exercise everyone enjoys, and it can be as gentle or as vigorous as you choose. It is anything but boring, because the number of dances that you can learn is endless.

Gardening

This is one of my personal favorites but is not for everyone. Mowing the lawn can be good exercise if you have the sort of mower that you walk behind, and digging, raking, and hoeing all provide good exercise. The main drawback is that a lot of the activities make you stoop, so watch your back!

How Much Training Is Needed?

A typical regimen would be one where you train for 30 minutes three or four times per week at about 70 percent of the maximum heart rate. This corresponds to a level at which you're not short of breath and can still carry on a conversation. You can estimate from Table 21.1 how much of each type of exercise you would need to burn off 1,500 calories per week.

An important point to be aware of is that the exercise does not have to be done all in one shot; it has been shown experimentally that three 10-minute bouts are as effective as one 30-minute bout.

SHOULD I JOIN A HEALTH CLUB?

Some people today seem to think that the only proper form of exercise is when you're wearing Lycra spandex and working out on a glossy black machine with a digital readout. There's nothing wrong with doing this, of course, and health clubs undoubtedly provide the greatest variety of exercise available. You can take a Walkman with you, and many of the clubs also have television. You can also meet friends there, and join in aerobics classes.

They are quite expensive, and they make their profits from people who sign on, pay their dues, and never go. My wife and I both belong to one, and part of the incentive for going is the sense of guilt engendered by knowing that we have paid all this money and shouldn't waste it!

SHOULD I MONITOR MY PULSE RATE DURING EXERCISE?

Some people get obsessional about what their pulse rate should be during exercise, but personally I never bother to check it. If you do want to find out what it is, you can stop exercising and then count it over 15 or 30 seconds, by feeling it either at the wrist (on the thumb side of the inside of the wrist joint) or in the neck (at the big carotid arteries on either side of your Adam's apple).

The official recommendation of the United States Preventive Services Task Force is that the pulse rate during training exercise should be 220 minus your age, multiplied by 70 percent. The rationale for this is that the maximum heart rate that you can achieve goes down with age (220 minus age is the formula for the maximum rate), and the recommendation is to exercise at 70 percent of maximum. This is a moderate level of exercise. The corresponding rates for different age groups are shown in Table 21.2.

**Table 21.2. Recommended Pulse Rates During
Exercise According to Age**

AGE	PULSE RATE
20	140/min
30	133/min
40	126/min
50	119/min
60	112/min
70	105/min

I should emphasize, however, that these numbers are only approximate, because people vary a lot in their maximum heart rates, so don't get too hung up on this subject. A better general guide is that you should exercise at an intensity at which you can still carry on a conversation with someone.

DOES IT MATTER IF I'M TAKING MEDICATIONS?

Unless your hypertension is very mild, you are probably taking blood-pressure-lowering medications. In fact, most doctors would recommend that you start an exercise program only after your pressure has been brought under reasonable control—for example, below 160/100 mm Hg. Most of the medications used to lower blood pressure should not affect your ability to exercise, with the exception of the beta blockers. These will limit the increase of systolic pressure during exercise (a good thing), and also the pumping ability of your heart (not necessarily such a good thing). What this means in practice is that at near-maximal levels of exercise your muscles may feel more tired than they otherwise would, but at lower levels you probably won't notice any difference. If you monitor your pulse after exercise, it's important to realize that it will always be slower if you're taking a beta blocker.

DOES THE TIME OF DAY AT WHICH I EXERCISE MATTER?

When you exercise is very much a matter of personal choice. Some people, like me, are morning people, and like to do it first thing in the morning. Others find it relaxing to do it in the evening when they get home from work. Some people are concerned that exercise is more dangerous in the morning than in the evening, because strokes and heart attacks are commoner then, but there's absolutely no evidence that this is related to people's exercise habits.

MAKING EXERCISE A PART OF YOUR LIFE

The important thing about exercise is that you need to keep on doing it. Dr. Ralph Paffenbarger's study of Harvard alumni showed that men who had been varsity athletes fared no better than their more sedentary colleagues in later life if they did not maintain their exercise habits. So it has to become part of your daily ritual, like brushing your teeth. This doesn't mean that you have to do it *every* day, but most people who do it regularly have a set time to do it.

SUMMARY

• A regular aerobic exercise program has numerous benefits: it will probably lower your blood pressure, help keep your weight down, reduce your chances of getting diabetes, heart disease, and osteoporosis, and help you cope with the effects of aging.

• Unless your pressure is way out of control, high blood pressure is not a reason for avoiding exercise.

• Choose the type of exercise that you enjoy most (or dislike least!) and that you can do on a regular basis.

• Three or four days a week for half an hour each time should be sufficient to get most of the benefits.

• If you get bored, do it in front of the TV or get a Walkman.

• Just do it!

CHAPTER TWENTY-TWO

BLOOD-PRESSURE-LOWERING MEDICATION

It used to be said of high blood pressure that the treatment was worse than the disease. This, of course, was because the condition itself is usually without symptoms, while many of the earlier forms of medication produced unpleasant side effects, such as impotence, diarrhea, and depression. Fortunately, things have got a lot better, and it's almost always possible to achieve adequate control of blood pressure without associated side effects. There is now a bewildering array of different medications available, and in this chapter we'll review how they work and what you should know about them.

THE REASONS FOR TAKING MEDICATION

Most of the medicines that we take are supposed to make us feel better—aspirin for relieving aches and pains, and antibiotics for treating infections, are two examples. With high blood pressure the situation is quite different: since most people have no symptoms to begin with, there is no prospect of feeling better as a result of taking blood-pressure-lowering medication. The reason for taking medication is also not simply to lower blood pressure, but to prevent its long-term consequences, such as strokes and heart attacks. Since blood pressure is a major risk factor for these conditions, it might seem reasonable to suppose that lowering it would automatically reverse the risk. However, this does not necessarily follow. All medications have side effects, and it is quite possible that some of these might cancel out the benefits derived from lowering the blood pressure.

WHAT ARE THE BENEFITS OF TAKING MEDICATION?

The first conclusive evidence that taking blood-pressure-lowering medication reduced the risks associated with high blood pressure was provided by the Veterans Administration study, which showed that treatment with diuretics and other drugs almost halved the risks. The subjects in this study were all male veterans, and they all had quite severe hypertension: to get into the study their diastolic pressure had to be at least 114 mm Hg. While this result was most encouraging, it left unanswered the question whether people with milder degrees of hypertension would also benefit from treatment, and whether women would fare as well as men. Since that time several other studies have helped to provide the answers.

One that attracted a lot of attention was the Hypertension Detection and Follow-up Program (HDFP), which was conducted in more than 10,000 patients, most of whom had diastolic pressures between 90 and 104 mm Hg at the start of the study. Half of the patients were allocated to the "stepped-care" group and were given blood-pressure-lowering medication in a series of steps designed to bring the pressure to below 90 mm Hg, while the other half were allocated to the "referred-care" group and were referred back to their doctors for less aggressive treatment. At the end of the five-year period of study the patients in the stepped-care group had diastolic pressures 5 mm Hg lower than the ones in the referred-care group, and nearly 20 percent fewer deaths. While this outcome was very encouraging, there are two major limitations. First, there was no benefit from treating white women, and second, there was no reduction in the number of heart attacks.

THE DOWNSIDE OF MEDICATION—COSTS AND SIDE EFFECTS

The above considerations show that it is clearly established that lowering high blood pressure with medication is generally beneficial, but there are also costs to be paid. One is financial, and the other is the side effects from the medication. The latter are of two general sorts: those arising from the normal actions of the drug, which depend on the dose, and those that occur as a result of some sort of allergic reaction. Some of these side effects, such as fatigue or impotence, may be noticed by the patient, while others, such as an elevation of the blood cholesterol level, can be detected only by blood tests.

THE TRADE-OFF BETWEEN THE COSTS AND BENEFITS OF TREATMENT

For your doctor to decide that your blood pressure should be treated with medication is often not an easy thing. It involves a judicious balancing of the advantages and disadvantages of treatment by comparing the relative weights of a number of factors. First is an assessment of your risk untreated. Obviously, the higher this is, the more urgent the need for treatment. This assessment should include a consideration of other risk factors as well as blood pressure. Next is the extent to which this risk can be reduced by treatment. Third are the cost and probability of side effects of treatment.

HOW YOUR DOCTOR CHOOSES YOUR MEDICATION

There are six or seven major classes of blood-pressure-lowering medications, each of which includes up to 20 individual agents. So how does your doctor choose the right one for you? It would be very satisfying to be able to say that he or she can tell which one will work best and with fewer, less troublesome side effects, but unfortunately this is not the case. There are some medications that cannot or should not be given to you if you have certain medical conditions: beta blockers, for example, make asthma worse. Beyond that, much of it is hit or miss.

HOW BLOOD-PRESSURE-LOWERING MEDICATIONS WORK

As we saw in Chapter 1, the basic problem in high blood pressure is that the arteries are constricted. A secondary cause is that the vascular system is overfilled, and the heart is pumping too much blood. Most of the blood-pressure-lowering medications work by opening up the constricted arteries, but they do so by a number of different mechanisms. Others, such as diuretics, work by reducing the volume of blood filling the system.

DIURETICS—TRADITIONAL FIRST-CHOICE AGENTS

For many years these agents, also referred to as water pills, have been the mainstay of antihypertensive treatment, and they have been used in all the clinical trials that have provided the evidence that treatment of hypertension can prevent the complications that result from it. Today, although they are still widely used, and by far the cheapest agents, their popularity is waning, partly because of genuine concerns about their safety, but also because of promotion by pharmaceutical companies of newer and more profitable agents.

How They Work. Diuretics work by preventing the reabsorption of salt and water from the urine while it is being formed in the kidneys. Consequently the volume of urine increases, and the amount of salt and water in the body is correspondingly reduced. They thus produce similar effects to going on a low-salt diet.

Every disturbance to the body's equilibrium provokes a reaction, and in the case of diuretics, the depletion of salt stimulates the kidneys to secrete renin, the end result of which is to increase the amount of aldosterone, a hormone that causes the kidney to retain sodium in exchange for potassium. If this reaction is very strong, as in people with an active renin system, the net effect of the diuretic on salt balance will be less than if it is weak, as occurs in people with "low-renin" hypertension. This explains why diuretics are more effective for lowering blood pressure in low-renin patients. It also explains why diuretics tend to cause depletion of potassium as well as of sodium.

Most diuretics make the kidneys lose potassium as well as sodium, which is generally not a good thing. There are, however, some that do not, and these are referred to as the potassium-retaining diuretics. They act on a different part of the kidney tubules where the urine is formed. The reason that they are not used more is that they are not as strong as the others, and their greatest use is in combination with the other diuretic agents.

Side Effects. The side effects of diuretics are of two sorts: ones that the patient notices, and metabolic effects that cause no symptoms but show up in your blood tests.

- *Increased Urination.* This, of course, is the mechanism by which diuretics work and is not strictly a side effect. It is usually less noticeable once you have been taking them for some time. It's one reason why diuretics are not taken at night.
- *Impotence.* This is one of the commoner side effects.
- *Gout.* If you develop an acute pain and swelling in your foot or ankle while taking a diuretic, the chances are that you have gout. It happens when uric acid, a waste product present in the blood, ac-

cumulates in a joint and crystallizes, thereby inflaming the joint. Diuretics interfere with the excretion of uric acid by the kidneys, and hence raise the blood levels.

- *Low Potassium.* The technical name for this is hypokalemia. Most diuretics lower the blood potassium level a little, but usually it's not enough to cause a problem. If extreme, it can cause muscle weakness, but although weakness while on a diuretic occurs, it's usually not from potassium depletion. A potentially more serious consequence of the low potassium is an instability of the rhythm of the heart (arrhythmia). Usually this takes the form of premature beats, which may be noticeable as skipped beats or palpitations, which are harmless, but occasionally a burst of several of them together can occur, which could be dangerous.
- *Low Magnesium.* This effect is usually only marginal, but it can contribute to the development of cardiac irregularities.
- *Increased Blood Sugar.* In a small proportion of people, diuretics may actually hasten the development of diabetes.
- *Increased Blood Cholesterol.* People who take diuretics for long periods may experience a subtle increase in their cholesterol levels, but if it occurs, it's usually only by a few points.

Some of the more commonly used diuretics are listed in Table 22.1.

Table 22.1. Some Commonly Used Diuretics

CLASS	BRAND NAME	GENERIC NAME
Thiazides	HydroDIURIL	Hydrochlorothiazide (HCTZ)
Loop diuretics	Lasix	Furosemide
Potassium-sparing diuretics	Aldactone	Spironolactone
	Midamor	Amiloride hydrochloride
Combination diuretics	Dyazide	HCTZ/Amiloride hydrochloride
	Maxzide	

ARE DIURETICS LESS SAFE THAN OTHER MEDICATIONS?

Diuretics have got a lot of bad press in the past few years, mainly because of concern about their metabolic side effects, particularly the changes of blood potassium, sugar, and cholesterol. There have also been claims that they may increase the risk of sudden death in people with heart disease. The dispute was stimulated by the findings of several large clinical trials of the effects of treating hypertension, which showed that while lowering the blood pressure had a dramatic effect on reducing strokes (by nearly half), the reduction of heart attacks was much less (by about 10 percent). Most of these studies used diuretics as the mainstay of treatment, prompting the question whether their beneficial effect on blood pressure might be offset by some of their other effects. If you improve one risk factor for heart disease (blood pressure) while at the same time worsening another (cholesterol), you might end up with no net benefit. In practice this is generally thought not to be a major concern, because the changes of cholesterol during long-term treatment with diuretics are very small, and theoretically not big enough to offset their beneficial effects on blood pressure.

The concern about the arrhythmia-producing effect of low potassium was fueled by some unexpected findings from the MRFIT study (Multiple Risk Factor Intervention Trial) that a subgroup of men with abnormal electrocardiograms who were treated with a diuretic had an increased mortality.

The proof of the pudding is in the eating, and when the results of all the major treatment trials are looked at closely the argument that diuretics increase the risk of heart attacks does not stand up. In the Medical Research Council Trial conducted in England, 2,213 patients received placebo treatment, and 1,081 a diuretic. There were 17.5 cardiovascular events per 1,000 patient-years in the group given diuretics, and 25.2 in the placebo group, showing that it was safer to take the diuretic.

Beta Blockers—Better Protection for the Heart?

The beta blockers are the other major group of blood-pressure-lowering medications that have been used in the major clinical trials. There's also a big debate going on about their effectiveness, but in this case it has to do with whether they are more effective than other types of medication at preventing heart attacks. One of the interesting things about them is that they were originally developed for treating heart disease (by Sir James Black, who was awarded a Nobel Prize for his work), and their effect on blood pressure was noticed only later.

How They Work. Beta blockers derive their name from the fact that they block beta receptors. The sympathetic nervous system, which regulates the actions of the heart and blood vessels, exerts its effects by secreting a chemical, norepinephrine, from nerve endings, which interacts with two main types of receptor (alpha and beta receptors) on the surfaces of the cells of the heart and blood vessels, and makes them contract or relax. Beta blockers sit on the beta receptors and prevent the norepinephrine from getting to them. Your heart rate is controlled by the sympathetic nervous system via beta receptors, and one of the most noticeable effects of beta blockers is that they slow the heart, particularly during exercise. They also reduce the pumping of the heart (cardiac output), which may be one mechanism by which they lower blood pressure, but a more important one is that they also inhibit renin secretion by the kidney. This explains why they tend to work best in people who have high-renin hypertension.

Because they stop the heart from working too hard, they are very useful in patients who have angina. This, in fact, was the condition for which they were originally developed, and their blood-pressure-lowering effect was discovered only incidentally.

Side Effects. The most noticeable side effect of beta blockers is fatigue, which stems from the lowered cardiac output. Thus, if you're physically very active, beta blockers may not be the best choice for you. Another effect is that they can cause slight constriction of the airways going to the lungs, which is not noticeable to most people, but means that they should not be given to people who have asthma.

The most widely used beta blockers are shown in Table 22.2.

Table 22.2. Commonly Used Beta Blockers

BRAND NAME	GENERIC NAME
Inderal	Propranolol hydrochloride
Corgard	Nadolol
Toprol, Lopressor	Metoprolol
Tenormin	Atenolol
Sectral	Acebutolol

ALPHA BLOCKERS—TWO BIRDS WITH ONE STONE?

Since high blood pressure and high blood cholesterol often coexist and interact to increase the risk of a heart attack, a medication that lowers both sounds like a gift from heaven. This claim has been made for the alpha blockers.

How They Work. Alpha blockers act by preventing the constriction of arteries produced by the sympathetic nervous system. In the same way that beta blockers sit on beta receptors, they block the alpha receptors on the muscle cells of the arteries, which are normally stimulated by norepinephrine to make the muscles contract. This opening up of the arteries lowers the blood pressure.

Side Effects. The very first dose of an alpha blocker can sometimes produce a dramatic reduction in blood pressure that is not seen with subsequent doses (sometimes referred to as a first-dose effect). This reduction in blood pressure may be particularly pronounced while you are standing, and make you feel faint. The problem can be avoided in two ways: first, by starting off with a very small dose and gradually increasing it, and second, by taking the medication at night, so that the peak effect occurs while you're in bed and less vulnerable to the effects of a sudden reduction in pressure. Other side effects include a stuffy nose and a skin rash.

The currently available alpha blockers are shown in Table 22.3.

Table 22.3. Alpha Blockers

BRAND NAME	GENERIC NAME
Minipress	Prazosin hydrochloride
Hytrin	Terazosin hydrochloride
Cardura	Doxazosin hydrochloride

CENTRALLY ACTING AGENTS

This class of drugs is not as popular as it used to be, because the side effects are more pronounced than with some of the other types. They lower blood pressure by a direct effect on the brain and, since the control of blood pressure and arousal are closely linked, tend to make people drowsy. The best known of these drugs is clonidine hydrochloride, which has recently been given a new lease on life by being made available as a skin patch, like a Band-Aid. One of these patches will work for about a week, which makes life a lot simpler than having to take pills two or three times a day. The patches also seem to be associated with somewhat fewer side effects than the pills.

How They Work. The sympathetic nervous system, which regulates the heart and blood vessels, originates in the brain (sometimes referred to as the central nervous system), and the centrally acting agents bind to receptors of brain cells whose function is to turn down the activity of the sympathetic nervous system, thereby lowering the blood pressure.

Side Effects. The most troublesome side effects are drowsiness and a dry mouth. These tend to lessen with time, but have limited the usefulness of these drugs.

Table 22.4 shows the centrally acting agents.

Table 22.4. Centrally Acting Agents

Brand Name	Generic Name
Catapres	Clonidine hydrochloride
Wytensin	Guanabenz acetate

Angiotensin Converting Enzyme Inhibitors (ACE Inhibitors)

This is one of the newer classes of blood-pressure-lowering agents and is rapidly growing in popularity. The ACE inhibitors, as they are commonly known, were designed specifically to block the effects of the renin-angiotensin system, which is one of the two major supports of the blood pressure. They work best in people who have high-renin hypertension, as you might expect. One reason for their popularity is that they don't produce the feelings of fatigue and listlessness that some of the other agents do.

How They Work. Angiotensin converting enzyme is a protein that triggers the conversion of angiotensin I, an inert substance, to angiotensin II, which is a highly potent constrictor of arteries. ACE inhibitors inactivate this enzyme and hence reduce the amount of angiotensin II in the bloodstream. This makes the arteries dilate and lowers the blood pressure. Their effectiveness, however, will clearly depend on how much angiotensin II there is to begin with. Since angiotensin production depends on the amount of renin present, this explains why ACE inhibitors work best in patients who have high-renin hypertension.

Side Effects. One of the selling points of ACE inhibitors has been that they do not produce the same feeling of fatigue that is seen with some of the other types of agent. While this has to some extent been supported by scientific studies, no drugs are perfect, and the ACE inhibitors are no exception. One of their most persistent side effects is a dry cough, which seems to be a characteristic of all the members of this class, although it affects only a small number of patients. The most serious side effect, which is fortunately extremely rare, is a swelling of the face and tongue. Others include loss of taste and skin rash.

The ACE inhibitors are listed in Table 22.5.

Table 22.5. Angiotensin Converting Enzyme
(ACE) Inhibitors

BRAND NAME	GENERIC NAME
Capoten	Captopril
Vasotec	Enalaprilat
Zestril	Lisinopril
Altace	Ramipril
Accupril	Quinapril
Lotensin	Benazepril
Monopril	Fosinopril

ANGIOTENSIN BLOCKING AGENTS

The newest type of antihypertensive drug is the angiotensin blocking agents, also referred to as AT I receptor blockers. The first of these to be approved was losartan, sold under the brand name Cozaar and in combination with a diuretic as Hyzaar. They are first cousins of the ACE inhibitors and work in a similar way, by blocking the effects of angiotensin, which constricts blood vessels and hence raises the pressure. But while the ACE inhibitors block the formation of angiotensin, the angiotensin antagonists block the receptors on the muscle cells that trigger its effects, and hence inactivate it.

It is too early to say exactly what the role of these agents will be, but they appear to be as effective as ACE inhibitors in controlling blood pressure and are well tolerated. One particular advantage over the ACE inhibitors is that they don't make you cough.

CALCIUM-CHANNEL BLOCKERS (CALCIUM ANTAGONISTS)

The contraction of the muscle cells of arteries is triggered by calcium entering the cell, which it does through special channels in the cell membrane known as calcium channels. As their name implies, calcium-channel blockers plug the entrance of these channels and weaken the contraction of the muscle cell. This relaxation dilates the artery and lowers the blood pressure. The contraction of heart muscle is also calcium-dependent, but the configuration of the channels is slightly different, so that some of the calcium-channel blockers have effects on the heart, while others do not. Calcium is not involved in the contraction of skeletal muscle cells, so they do not produce any muscle weakness. Their ability to dilate coronary arteries accounts for their effectiveness in angina as well as in hypertension.

Side Effects. Some of the side effects of calcium-channel blockers are due to their physiological actions. Constipation is one example, which is noticed by some people while taking verapamil, and occurs because the drug tends to inhibit the contraction of the muscles of the intestines. Another is swelling of the ankles, which is seen with several calcium-channel blockers and is attributable to the dilation of small blood vessels, causing them to leak fluid into the tissues. Ankle swelling is often a sign of fluid retention, but in this particular case it has a quite different explanation. Rather than causing retention of fluid, calcium-channel blockers have a slight diuretic effect—that is, they cause an overall reduction of the amount of salt and water in the body.

The calcium-channel blockers are shown in Table 22.6.

Table 22.6. Calcium-Channel Blockers

BRAND NAME	GENERIC NAME
Procardia	Nifedipine
Calan, Isoptin, Verelan	Verapamil hydrochloride
Cardizem, Dilacor	Diltiazem hydrochloride
Plendil	Felodipine
Norvasc	Amlodipine
DynaCirc	Isradipine

Are Calcium-Channel Blockers Less Safe than Other Blood-Pressure-Lowering Drugs?

Calcium-channel blockers have recently come under fire as first-line agents for the treatment of high blood pressure, mainly as a result of two studies which were published in the summer of 1995. The first was a retrospective study conducted in a managed care organization in Seattle that claimed that patients who were having their blood pressure treated by calcium-channel blockers had a 60 percent higher risk of having a heart attack than those being treated with other drugs, particularly when the drugs were given in high doses. While these figures are disturbing, they are unconfirmed and should be regarded with some skepticism, because the analysis was conducted retrospectively, and it is not clear why those particular patients were prescribed calcium-channel blockers in the first place. A plausible explanation is that their doctors thought (correctly) that they already had heart disease, and chose calcium-channel blockers on the grounds that they might prevent the consequences.

The second study was an analysis of sixteen randomized trials in which nifedipine (the generic name of Procardia, the most widely used calcium-channel blocker) was compared with a placebo in patients who were recovering from a heart attack. The objective of the trials was to see if the nifedipine would prevent a second heart attack. The analysis showed that if the nifedipine was given in small doses (80 mg a day or less), it had no effect one way or the other. But when given in high doses (more than 80 mg) it increased the risk of a second heart attack nearly threefold.

The interpretation of these findings has aroused much controversy. At the time at which these studies were done, nifedipine was available only in its original formulation, which is very short-acting. It lowers blood pressure within 30 minutes and its effects wear off within three or four hours. Nowadays it is also available in an extended-release form that produces a gentle and steady reduction of blood pressure, so that it needs to be taken only once a day. The other calcium-channel blockers also have a less violent action than short-acting nifedipine.

The National Heart, Lung, and Blood Institute reviewed these data and issued a warning statement about nifedipine, with which I would agree. It can be summarized as follows:

- Short-acting nifedipine (available as Procardia or Adalat capsules in 10- and 20-mg doses) should not be used for long-term blood pressure reduction.
- There is no evidence for any adverse effects of the long-acting (extended-release) forms of nifedipine such as Procardia XL or Adalat CC, which are available as tablets of 30, 60, or 90 milligrams.
- There is no evidence for any major adverse effects of the other calcium-channel blockers.

Ultimately, the question as to the safety of calcium-channel blockers can be settled only by a randomized controlled trial, which is in fact now being conducted. In the meantime, what should you do if you're taking one of these drugs? I still prescribe them for my own patients, although they are not my first choice. There are many patients in whom calcium-channel blockers control blood pressure better and with milder side effects than other types of drugs, and if you're one of these, don't switch. You may want to discuss the issue with your doctor.

VASODILATORS

These agents are used only for problem cases in which the blood pressure cannot be controlled by the types of drugs described above. The reason for this is that when used on their own they produce an increased heart rate and fluid retention, which means that they are best given in combination with other agents that combat these effects.

How They Work. The vasodilators act directly on the arterial muscle cells to relax them and hence to dilate the artery and lower blood pressure. This effect is independent of the renin-angiotensin and sympathetic nervous systems, which are stimulated reflexly by the fall of blood pressure to oppose the effect of the vasodilator and to maintain the blood pressure at its original level.

DOES IT MATTER WHEN I TAKE MY MEDICATIONS?

Nowadays, most blood-pressure-lowering medications need to be taken only once a day. In some cases this is because the medications are naturally long-acting, and in others because they are packaged as slow-release preparations. The goal is to lower the blood pressure throughout the day and night, and when the FDA approves a new drug it requires proof that this is achieved with the recommended dosing schedule. A medication that is recommended for dosing once a day typically starts to work about 1 or 2 hours after it's swallowed, and exerts its maximum effect at about 4 to 6 hours. After that the effect gradually wears off.

Most people take their medications first thing in the morning, but most once-a-day medications can also be taken at night. You might think that since most medications have their maximum effect about 4 to 6 hours after you take them, they might lower the blood pressure too much during the night if you take them just before you go to bed. In fact, this doesn't seem to be a problem; we performed a study of one of these long-acting medications taken at night and monitored the changes of pressure with an ambulatory monitor. Somewhat to our surprise, we found that the peak effect on the blood pressure occurred during the following morning, when of course the pressure is normally at its highest. So taking the medication at night makes a lot of sense.

The important thing is to choose a time that makes it easy to remember to take the medications every day. Usually this means at the time of getting up, going to bed, or meals.

WILL I EVENTUALLY DEVELOP IMMUNITY TO THE EFFECTS OF THE MEDICATION?

Most medications work for an indefinite length of time, so if yours is working, there's no reason to suppose that it won't continue to do so.

WHY ARE SOME MEDICATIONS SO EXPENSIVE?

One of the things that you will very soon notice if you're having to take medication is the enormous variation in the price. Some, like hydrochlorothiazide, cost virtually nothing, while others, like some of the newer ACE inhibitors, may cost as much as $1 for one pill. How are the prices regulated? In the United States the answer is very simple—the pharmaceutical manufacturers control them. According to the Pharmaceutical Manufacturers Association, which is a powerful lobbying group for the industry, it costs $231 million to bring one new prescription drug to the market. An independent analysis by Stephen Schondelmeyer, an economist at the University of Minnesota, concluded that only 16 percent of a drug's cost is attributable to research and development, while 22 percent goes to marketing costs.

You might think that because there is a lot of competition among drug companies for market share, there would be an incentive to keep prices down. Unfortunately for the consumer, this is not what happens. As is the case with health care in general, the normal market forces are very distorted. The pharmaceutical companies aim their marketing almost exclusively at doctors, not at patients, and while the doctors write the prescriptions, it is the patients who pay the bills. When a new class of drug is introduced, it's not unreasonable to expect that the first drug of that class will be expensive, because of the development costs. However, most of the drugs that are approved by the FDA are "me too" drugs, which are simply variations on a theme. You would think that they would be cheaper, both because they cost less to develop and because the companies introducing them would want to increase their market share by competitive pricing. This doesn't happen, partly because doctors are generally insensitive to the prices of medications, and in my experience patients rarely ask about comparative prices of medications. A classic example was the blockbuster anti–stomach ulcer medicine called Tagamet. For six years it was the only drug of its class, and it made millions of dollars of profit for SmithKline. But when the second drug, Zantac, was introduced by Glaxo in direct competition, it was not priced any lower than Tagamet, and neither was the price of Tagamet reduced. Subsequently two other drug companies (Lilly and Merck) introduced their own ulcer drugs, both priced a little higher than Tagamet. Thus, while drug companies certainly do compete with one another, they rarely do so by price cutting.

The way they do compete is by marketing to doctors. This is done partly by advertisements in medical journals, but far more persuasive are the sales representatives, whose job it is to frequent doctors' offices and talk to the doctors about their products. In our institution they also provide free lunches for the cardiologists in training. There are 45,000 representatives in the United States (one for every twelve doctors), and the average doctor sees two or three a week. They typically leave free samples of medication as well as promotional literature. The importance of these samples is that the doctor uses them to start the patient on the new medication, and everyone is happy for a while—until the patient has to pay for the next prescription.

There is, however, an enormous range of prices charged by pharmacies. A survey conducted by the New York City Department of Consumer Affairs found that someone living in Manhattan might be paying $47.76 for blood pressure medication that cost $25.50 in Queens. Some of their findings are shown in Table 22.7.

Table 22.7. Range of Prices of Drugs in New York City Drugstores

DRUG	DOSE	NUMBER OF PILLS	HIGH	LOW	% DIFFERENCE
Calan	80 mg	60	$49.95	$22.95	118
generic	80 mg	60	$39.95	$ 7.75	415
Capoten	25 mg	60	$71.15	$31.95	123
Cardizem	30 mg	60	$49.95	$20.45	144
Dyazide	—	30	$27.95	$ 9.37	198
Lanoxin	0.25 mg	100	$39.95	$ 5.37	644
Procardia	10 mg	90	$90.63	$38.38	136
Tenormin	50 mg	30	$49.95	$22.59	121
generic	50 mg	30	$31.39	$ 9.29	238
Vasotec	10 mg	60	$97.13	$32.50	199

Drug prices are generally higher in the United States than in most other countries, because in most countries there is some form of government regulation. In Canada, the Patent Medicine Prices Review Board has the power to remove patent protection from drugs that it considers too expensive. As a result, drug prices are on average 30 percent lower than in the United States.

Most other countries have some form of governmental regulation of drug prices, either direct or indirect. According to Jean-Pierre Poullier, a medical economist working for the Organization for Economic Cooperation and Development, American drug prices are among the highest of the 24 OECD nations, and have also been rising faster than any other's.

Things are likely to change in the United States in the near future. As part of their program of health care reform, members of the Clinton administration are looking into the possibility of regulating drug prices in the United States, along the lines of the Canadian system, and Representative Pete Stark of California has introduced a bill to establish a regulatory board. The drug companies are naturally opposed to any such scheme but are beginning to get the message. Merck recently proposed a voluntary system of price restraints, under which the average rate of increase in drug prices would not exceed the rate of inflation. And the drug companies may be starting to compete with one another on price. Advertisements for drugs in medical journals virtually never mention cost, but recently Miles placed a six-page ad for a long-acting preparation of nifedipine called Adalat CC whose theme was its 25 percent lower cost in comparison with Procardia XL, Pfizer's hugely successful version of nifedipine, resulting in annual savings to the consumer of $111 to $217.

SHOULD I TAKE GENERIC DRUGS?

It is well known that generic drugs are a lot cheaper than brand-name versions, and it's been estimated that the average saving per prescription by using generics is $7.50. But a lot of people are concerned that the generics are not the same as the original brand-name drug. For many of the antihypertensive drugs commonly used, there is no choice: the patent lasts for 17 years, and until it runs out there will be no generic. So one thing you can be sure about is that if you are prescribed a generic drug it's tried and true. There is a long list of brand-name drugs that had to be hurriedly withdrawn before they were available as generics after it was discovered that they had previously undetected serious side effects.

In 1984 Congress passed the Drug Price Competition and Patent Term Restoration Act, which provided for expedited approval of generic drugs. This mandated that the testing of a generic be confined to measuring drug levels in healthy volunteers. All that is needed is to establish that the generic form is chemically identical with the brand-name version and that it is absorbed as well into the body. There should be no need to do extensive testing for side effects, since this will already have been done for the brand-name version. The FDA requires that the generics meet the same standards of strength, quality, and purity as the brand-name product.

The passing of the 1984 act had the expected effect. Within three years after a generic version of a drug came on the market, the sales of the brand-name version fell on average by 50 percent. The brand-name companies made no attempt to reduce their prices to compete, and in fact a study sponsored by the Health Care Financing Administration showed that the annual rate of price increase after 1984 was four times greater for brand-name versions than for generics.

The other policy that the makers of brand-name medications have adopted is "if you can't lick 'em, join 'em." In Puerto Rico, where for tax reasons a large proportion of drugs are manufactured, SmithKline Beecham makes Dyazide, a popular diuretic. The medicine is manufactured in a perfectly uniform way but is packaged in two types of capsules. Some are red and maroon, and are sold as Dyazide by SmithKline at $35.20 per 100, while others are white, and are sold by a subsidiary firm called Rugby as hydrochlorothiazide plus triamterene (a much less catchy name) at $25.24. Another very successful antihypertensive drug, marketed by its discoverer ICI (now known as Zeneca) as Tenormin (generic name atenolol) at $80.20 per 100, is also available at $65.02 in generic form from a company called IPR, and at $45.25 from Goldline. What most people do not realize is that all three preparations are manufactured in the same factory in Puerto Rico, and all the companies are controlled by Zeneca.

CAN I EVER GET OFF THE MEDICATIONS ONCE I START?

This is a common concern, but the good news is that taking blood-pressure-lowering medication is not a life sentence. With many of my patients I try gradually withdrawing the medication if the blood pressure is normal for several months, and sometimes we succeed, without the blood pressure going up.

SUMMARY

- The reason for taking blood-pressure-lowering medication is not to make you feel better, but to minimize your risk of having a stroke or heart attack.

- Not everyone needs to start taking medication at the same level of blood pressure—it depends on your overall level of risk.

- There's no single type of medication that is superior to any other; the trick is to find one that controls your pressure without giving you side effects.

- There's a huge variation in the costs of medications, depending on what they are and where you buy them. The more expensive ones are not necessarily better.

- Generics are always cheaper and generally no less effective than the equivalent brand-name product.

- It's not true that once you start on blood-pressure-lowering medication you'll never be able to get off it.

CHAPTER TWENTY-THREE

CHOLESTEROL-LOWERING MEDICATION

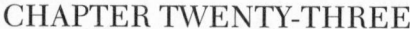

Although the primary focus of this book is on high blood pressure and its treatment, high blood cholesterol is commonly associated with it; and to an increasing extent, people are prescribed medications to lower both blood pressure and cholesterol. In the United States and elsewhere, the use of cholesterol-lowering agents is one of the fastest-growing sectors of the pharmaceutical industry. While dietary change is recommended as a first step for lowering cholesterol and triglycerides, many people are disappointed with the results (see Chapter 18), which raises the question of whether they should start to take medication. We have already seen that there is considerable uncertainty as to exactly when blood-pressure-lowering medication should be started, but with cholesterol the situation is even less clear. Effective medications have been available for a much shorter period of time, and studies of their long-term efficacy are few and far between. There is no doubt that they can lower blood cholesterol and triglyceride levels, but whether this will eventually translate into fewer deaths from heart disease remains, for many of them, unproven. In fact, the biggest controversy at the moment centers on the possibility that the benefits from fewer heart disease deaths are offset by increased deaths from other causes, as discussed below.

Do Cholesterol-lowering Drugs Reduce Deaths from Heart Disease?

The short answer to this question is "Yes, but." An ever increasing number of studies have been reported that have attempted to answer this question, and until recently, the general consensus was that they reduce the death rate from heart disease, but not the overall death rate. You don't have to be a rocket scientist to conclude that this means that they must increase the death rate from other causes. A good example of a study investigating this was the Finnish Heart Study in which men who had recovered from a heart attack were given a drug called gemfibrozil and compared with a similar number of men in a control group, who did not receive the drug. At the end of a five-year follow-up period the rate for recurrent heart attacks was 34 percent lower in the treatment group than in the controls.

A furious controversy subsequently arose concerning the apparent increase, in the treated group, of death from causes other than heart disease: Is it a chance finding or is it due to an adverse effect of the drugs? As other studies show, the problem is that such deaths do not appear to be associated with any one particular drug, or with any single cause of death. Whatever the explanation, the question keeps cropping up, and cannot lightly be dismissed.

One of the most illuminating analyses of the evidence was performed by Dr. George Davey Smith and his colleagues. They looked at 35 trials of the effects of cholesterol reduction, some of which relied on diet, and others on drugs. They divided these trials into three groups according to the level of risk of heart disease of the patients who were recruited into the studies. In the trials that recruited high-risk patients (for example, people who had already had a heart attack) there was clear evidence of benefit from the treatment, which lowered the mortality of the treated groups. In the medium-risk trials the result was a wash, but in the trials in which patients were at low risk to begin with, the treatment actually raised mortality.

When the trials were separated into those that used drugs and those that used diet, it became apparent that mortality from non–heart disease causes was increased only in the trials in which drugs were used to lower the cholesterol. The main implication of this analysis is that there is a benefit from lowering cholesterol in the form of a reduction of coronary heart disease, but also that there is a small risk associated with the use of the drugs, which manifests itself as death from other causes. In individuals who are at very high risk of heart disease, the benefits from taking drugs clearly outweigh the risks, but in low-risk individuals the drugs may do more harm than good.

One of the criticisms of these earlier trials was that they didn't include enough people to be sure that overall mortality was being affected by the treatment. This question has recently been laid to rest with the publication of what has been called the "4S," or Scandinavian Simvastatin Survival Study. There were 4,444 patients with heart disease (angina or a previous heart attack) and a high blood cholesterol despite being on a low-fat diet who were allocated to take either simvastatin (a cholesterol-lowering drug similar to lovastatin) or a placebo. After five and a half years the drug lowered the total cholesterol by 25 percent, the LDL cholesterol by 35 percent, and it raised the HDL by 8 percent, all of which were desirable effects. The big finding of the study was that 256 patients in the placebo group died, compared with only 182 in the sim-vastatin group—a 30 percent reduction in the death rate. The reduction in deaths from heart attacks was even more dramatic, and was close to 50 percent. Even more reassuringly, there was no excess of deaths from noncardiac causes in the treated group, as had been found in some of the earlier studies. The benefits of treatment were apparent in both men and women, and in older (i.e., over 60 years) as well as younger patients.

The very clear-cut results of this study confirm that if you already have heart disease and a high cholesterol, you should have your choles-terol lowered, if necessary by drugs. What the results do not say, how-ever, is that you should be taking the drugs if your cholesterol is normal to begin with, even if you do have heart disease, or that you should be taking them when you have a high cholesterol without any known heart problems. Those are more difficult decisions, and will need to be made in consultation with your doctor.

AT WHAT LEVEL OF CHOLESTEROL SHOULD MEDICATION BE STARTED?

The National Cholesterol Education Program (NCEP) has issued two sets of guidelines to answer this question, based on the level of LDL cho-lesterol and on whether there is evidence of existing heart disease. The first set, published in 1988, made strong recommendations for using drugs. It was subsequently pointed out that if these had been followed, up to 10 percent of the population would now be on cholesterol-lowering medication. The second set was published in 1993 and was much more selective. (The recommendations are described in Chapter 2.) They take into consideration the number of risk factors for heart disease other than a high cholesterol. Which category you fall into thus depends on (a) whether you've already been diagnosed as having coronary heart disease (CHD), and (b) how many risk factors you have. These are shown in Table 23.1.

Table 23.1. CHD Risk Factors Used to Decide Treatment for High Cholesterol (NCEP Guidelines)

Positive
*Age—Male over 45 years
*Female over 55, or premature menopause and not taking estrogens
*Family history of premature CHD (heart attack before age 55 years in father or before 65 in mother)
*Smokes cigarettes
*High blood pressure
*Low HDL cholesterol (below 35)
*Diabetes

Negative
*High HDL cholesterol (above 60)

Using this table you can work out how many risk factors you have; note that if your HDL is above 60 this will cancel out one of the other factors. If you know your LDL cholesterol level, you can then go to Table 23.2 to see what sort of treatment is recommended. (If you know only your total cholesterol, a level of 240 total corresponds to 160 LDL, and 200 total to 130 LDL.) The official policy is to start with the Step One diet for three months, and then if this doesn't work to go on to Step Two, and then if necessary to drugs.

Table 23.2. NCEP Guidelines for Diet and Drug Treatment of High LDL Cholesterol

PATIENT CATEGORY	INITIAL LDL	GOAL LDL
Start diet if . . .		
*No known CHD and fewer than 2 risk factors	Above 160	Below 160
*No known CHD and 2 or more risk factors	Above 130	Below 130
*Known to have CHD	Above 100	Below 100
Start drugs if . . .		
*No known CHD and fewer than 2 risk factors	Above 190	Below 160
*No known CHD and 2 or more risk factors	Above 160	Below 130
*Known to have CHD	Above 130	Below 100

The reason for the distinction between people with and without known heart disease is simple: on both theoretical and practical grounds, it makes more sense to be aggressive about lowering the cholesterol when we know that it's already caused a problem, as in the people with known heart disease, or if there's a high probability that it will do so, as in the people with three major risk factors (for example, high blood pressure and diabetes as well as a high cholesterol). In people without heart disease or with fewer risk factors, the chances that the high cholesterol will cause a problem are correspondingly lower.

MEDICATIONS USED TO LOWER CHOLESTEROL

There are now a number of different medications available to treat disorders of blood lipids, ranging from niacin, which is the original agent and a cheap over-the-counter vitamin, to the "statins," which are the newest group and quite expensive. We'll meet niacin again in the next chapter, and in this section will focus on the prescription medications.

Table 23.3 shows some of the main ones and their effects on blood lipids. Also included are the changes that can be achieved by diet alone; notice how much more potent the medications are.

Table 23.3. Effects of Different Cholesterol-lowering Drugs

| CLASS | DRUG* | EXPECTED EFFECT | | |
		LDL	HDL	TG†
Step One diet (30% fat)		– 5%	– 5%	
Step Two diet (30% fat)		–10%		
Step Three diet (20% fat)		–20%		
Nicotinic acid	Niacin	–20%	+25%	–40%
Bile acid sequestrants	Questran (cholestyramine)	–25%	+ 5%	0
	Colestid (colestipol hydrochloride)			
Fibric acid derivatives	Lopid (gemfibrozil)	–15%	+20%	–40%
Statins	Mevacor (lovastatin)			
	Zocor (simvastatin)	–30%	+ 5%	–10%
	Pravachol (pravastatin)			
Probucol	Lorelco (probucol)	–10%	–15%	0

*Drug names are listed as brand name with generic in parentheses.
†TG = triglycerides.

Niacin

Niacin is generally the first drug to be tried when diet alone doesn't do the trick. It has been used for much longer than any of the drugs described below, and was the first to be proven to be able to prevent heart disease. It's also one of the most potent, and produces changes in the desired direction of all the three major classes of lipids (see Table 23.3), which the other available drugs do not. Its big drawback is its side effects; to be fully effective it needs to be taken in quite large doses (up to 3 grams a day), and many people can't tolerate that amount.

Because it's not a prescription drug, it's described in Chapter 24.

Resins (Questran and Colestid)

These are powders that are normally taken with food and are not absorbed from the bowel. They act by mopping up bile acids, which are excreted by the liver into the bowel and then reabsorbed to be used in the synthesis of cholesterol. The powders have a gritty texture that is not pleasant, and they tend to make you constipated. They are packaged in various disguises designed to make them more palatable, with added flavoring or as candy bars. The powders can be mixed with cold drinks or food, but cannot be cooked with food, because that would inactivate them. They also interfere with the absorption of some other medications, which should therefore not be taken at the same time.

They are of proven efficacy, and have been shown not only to lower cholesterol but also to lower the rate of heart attacks in patients with high cholesterol levels.

Their chief disadvantage is that they have to be taken two or three times a day before meals, and many patients find them unpalatable.

Side Effects. The most common problems are various types of stomach upset, including indigestion, nausea, and constipation. Other less common side effects include weight loss, skin rash, and bruising.

Statins

The technical name of this group of drugs is HMG CoA reductase inhibitors. They get this rather indigestible title because their mode of action is to inhibit the action of an enzyme called HMG CoA reductase, which is involved in the synthesis of cholesterol by the liver. They are normally taken at night, because that is the time when cholesterol synthesis is at its maximum. The simpler term *statins* is sometimes used because the three currently approved agents in this class all have statin in their generic name (lovastatin, pravastatin, and simvastatin). They can produce a dramatic reduction in total and LDL cholesterol levels, with a smaller decrease in triglycerides and a slight increase in HDL. Their chief advantage is their low incidence of side effects in comparison with the other classes of lipid-lowering drugs.

The first member of this group to be introduced, lovastatin, has been shown to slow the progression of atherosclerosis in the coronary arteries in angiography studies. In one of these, called the MARS (Monitored Atherosclerosis Regression Study), 270 patients with documented coronary heart disease were randomly allocated to receive either placebo or lovastatin in a dose of 80 milligrams per day. At the end of two years the lovastatin had lowered the total cholesterol by 32 percent, the LDL by 38 percent, and the HDL was raised 8 percent. All the patients had a repeat angiogram. The results showed that plaques that blocked more than 50 percent of the arterial lumen decreased by 4 percent in the patients given lovastatin, and progressed by 1 percent in the patients given placebo. These differences may not seem very big, but they could be quite important if continued over many years. There were one third fewer coronary events in the group given lovastatin in the MARS, but the number of patients in the study was too small to know if this was a genuine effect of the drug.

It is now clear that the statins can also reduce heart attacks, as evidenced by the "4S" from Scandinavia, described above.

Side Effects. These are relatively rare, although it is not uncommon for increases in the blood levels of some liver enzymes to occur. The significance of this is not clear: it causes no symptoms, and is reversible if the drug is stopped. Most doctors recommend reducing the dose or discontinuing the drug when it occurs. Other side effects include muscle weakness, headaches, and insomnia.

Fibrates

This class of drugs is derived from fibric acid, which explains their name. The first one was clofibrate (Atromid), which is no longer used. It has been succeeded by gemfibrozil (Lopid), whose effectiveness in preventing heart attacks has been demonstrated in a large Finnish study. The chief effects of these drugs are to reduce triglycerides and to raise HDL. LDL cholesterol is lowered only a small amount. They are most appropriate for use in patients with very high cholesterol/HDL ratios, particularly when the HDL is low.

Side Effects. The main side effects are digestive in nature: indigestion, nausea, stomach pains, and flatulence. Others include muscle weakness, headache, and alterations in liver enzymes. They have to be used with caution when combined with other medications that affect liver and muscle enzymes, such as niacin and the statins.

Probucol

This drug was originally developed as a commercial antioxidant for industry, and was subsequently found to lower LDL cholesterol. It was then discovered that oxidation of cholesterol plays an important part in the development of atheroma, which renewed interest in probucol. As well as lowering LDL, it also lowers HDL, which of course is not what one would want. It remains to be seen whether probucol will actually prevent coronary heart disease. If it acts as an antioxidant, it might delay the formation of plaque without its effect being detected by any change in the blood lipids. A clinical trial is currently being conducted to see if it will have this effect.

Because its long-term benefits, if any, are unproven, and cannot be estimated from its rather meager effects on the blood lipids, I do not recommend probucol.

Side Effects. It may cause a slight change in the electrocardiogram, but this is not of any known consequence. Like other lipid-lowering agents, it can also cause stomach upsets, such as nausea, pain, and diarrhea.

CAN BLOOD-PRESSURE-LOWERING AND CHOLESTEROL-LOWERING DRUGS BE COMBINED?

Many people have both high blood pressure and high cholesterol, and increasingly their doctors are prescribing medications to lower both. Although there have been very few studies investigating whether the combinations are safe, there doesn't seem to be a problem. The only exception to this is the resins such as Questran, which can interfere with the absorption of other drugs.

COMPARATIVE COSTS OF CHOLESTEROL-LOWERING MEDICATIONS

One thing that distinguishes the different cholesterol medications is their cost. The comparative costs of the main different types for a year's treatment are shown in Table 23.4.

Table 23.4. Comparative Costs of Lipid-lowering Medications

DRUG	BRAND NAME	COST
Nicotinic acid	Niacin	$50–$200
Cholestyramine	Questran	$500
Gemfibrozil	Lopid	$600
Lovastatin	Mevacor	$500–$2,100

It is worth noting that tablets of all the statins come in two strengths, and that the cost of the greater dose is relatively less than for the smaller one. Thus pravastatin 10 milligrams costs about $1.53 per pill, while the 20-milligram pill is $1.80. Therefore, if you're on a big dose, it's important to make sure that you have the 20-milligram pills.

SUMMARY

• It's quite likely that you may not be able to control your cholesterol level by diet alone. There's no absolute level of cholesterol above which you should start taking medications to lower it—as with blood pressure it depends on your level of risk.

• Niacin is usually tried first, but may have side effects.

• The most powerful medications are the "statins."

CHAPTER TWENTY-FOUR

VITAMINS AND HEALTH FOODS

The past few years have witnessed a huge growth in the health-food industry, with the promotion of traditional herbal remedies and vitamins, packaged in pills by their promoters, as preventives and cures for just about every disease known to man, including even aging. In this chapter I will review how these agents can affect blood pressure and the risk of getting cardiovascular disease.

VITAMINS: FACTS AND FADS

Walk into any health-food store and you will be faced with shelves laden with assortments of vitamin pills, for which claims are made to cure all sorts of diseases, ranging from cancer to heart disease, and including the common cold and high blood pressure. The idea that vitamins can prevent disease has a long history, and dates back to 1753, when the Scottish naval surgeon James Lind showed that scurvy, a major cause of disability and death in sailors on long sea voyages, could be prevented by drinking the juice of lemons, limes, or oranges. It was subsequently shown that the crucial ingredient was ascorbic acid, or vitamin C. Other vitamins—chemical substances present in plants or animals, small amounts of which are essential for our health, and which our bodies cannot manufacture—were subsequently discovered. There are at least 13 of these substances altogether, most of which need not concern us here.

The traditional view of vitamins was that they are needed only in very small amounts, and that if people are eating a reasonably balanced diet, which includes a variety of foods such as fruits and vegetables, they don't need to worry. Vitamin deficiency is likely to occur only in people who eat a diet that is completely lacking in one or more food groups, such as the sailors who, before Lind's discovery, had no fruits or vegetables because they rotted during long voyages. In contemporary society overt vitamin deficiency is relatively uncommon, but does occur in people who are either malnourished or who eat fad diets.

The situation changed entirely when Dr. Linus Pauling, who had the unique scientific prestige of having won two Nobel Prizes, wrote a book in 1970 called *Vitamin C and the Common Cold,* in which he claimed that very large doses of vitamin C could prevent people from catching colds. The Recommended Daily Allowance (RDA) of vitamin C is 60 milligrams (the amount in 4 ounces of orange juice), but Dr. Pauling's recommendation was for 500 milligrams or more. He subsequently claimed that a dose of 10 grams a day could prolong survival in patients with terminal cancer. Despite the fact that neither of these claims has been substantiated in controlled clinical trials, Dr. Pauling's prestige was sufficient to usher in the era of megadoses of vitamins, in which it is assumed that more is necessarily better. Dr. Pauling also had other less publicized beliefs, however. In 1984 he served as a witness for the defense of a quack doctor who was accused of using unproven remedies to treat cancer. Dr. Pauling defended the use of megadoses not only of vitamin C but also of vitamin A (which can produce toxic effects) and of coffee enemas and chelation therapy (discussed in Chapter 27). Even Nobel Prize winners can be wrong.

The truth of the matter probably lies somewhere between the two extreme views—on the one hand that the RDA for all the vitamins is all that anyone needs, and on the other that everyone should be taking megadoses. The RDAs were originally defined as the minimum amount of a vitamin needed to prevent deficiency diseases: for vitamin C, scurvy; for vitamin A, pellagra; and for vitamin D, rickets. The result has been that these diseases are now very rare in westernized societies. Since that time, however, there has been an ever increasing body of evidence to indicate that several vitamins may play a role in retarding the development of chronic diseases such as cancer and heart disease. This evidence is of two kinds: epidemiological studies and studies of the disease processes in experimental animals. The most exciting part of this story is the role of certain vitamins (particularly beta-carotene, vitamin C, and vitamin E) as antioxidants.

FREE RADICALS AND ANTIOXIDANTS

The term *free radicals,* which sounds as though it might refer to political activists of the thirties, has become very fashionable lately, and *The New York Times* devoted an article to them in a recent supplement. They are in fact unstable chemicals that are normally present in our bodies and are thought to play a role in the development of heart disease and cancer. Technically, they are atoms or molecules with a single electron in their outer shell, which explains their unstable nature, since electrons normally go around in pairs. They are the normal by-products of metabolism, particularly of oxygen, but their formation can be increased by stimuli such as cigarette smoke and the cosmic radiation experienced on a cross-country plane trip.

Although oxygen is essential to human life, it is one of the major sources of free radicals. These may occur when the blood level of oxygen suddenly decreases and then increases (as, for example, would occur when there is a transient blockage of an artery). These radicals can cause serious damage to the delicate lining of the artery, but are normally mopped up by scavenging chemicals in the blood, known as antioxidants, of which vitamins C and E are two notable examples.

VITAMINS, VEGETABLES, AND DISEASE

The two major causes of death from chronic disease are heart disease and cancer. There is now epidemiological evidence from all over the world that the death rate from both may be related to a low intake of fruits and vegetables, and that the antioxidant vitamins may be some of the crucial ingredients that confer the beneficial effects.

VITAMIN C (ASCORBIC ACID)

There are several ways in which vitamin C may help to prevent heart disease. It has been known for at least 10 years that consuming 500 to 1,000 milligrams of vitamin C daily can lower total blood cholesterol levels by up to 10 percent. There's a catch to this, however, because it's likely to happen only if you're at least marginally deficient in vitamin C to begin with. If you're already consuming an adequate amount, taking more won't have much effect. Two groups of people who are likely to be marginally deficient are smokers and diabetics, both of which groups are at greater risk of heart disease. The recommended daily allowance is 50 to 100 milligrams, which is about the amount in one glass of orange juice.

Three large-scale health surveys have shown a relationship between blood levels of vitamin C and HDL cholesterol (the good kind). One study found that feeding 1,000 milligrams of vitamin C daily to a group of elderly people who were deficient in vitamin C raised their HDL levels, but three other studies done with younger and healthier people found no effect. The message here is the same as with the effect on total cholesterol: it's important to maintain an adequate level, but megadoses have no additional benefit.

There are also several population studies showing that higher blood levels of vitamin C are associated with lower blood pressure. This has been found in the United States, Finland, and Japan. It may merely reflect the fact that people who eat a healthy diet rich in fruits and vegetables tend to have lower blood pressure. Surprisingly, there has been no properly controlled study of the effects of feeding vitamin C to hypertensive subjects. About the only information we have is from one study of 27 elderly men and women in whom 400 milligrams per day of vitamin C taken for four weeks produced no consistent lowering of blood pressure. This is clearly an area that deserves further study.

Sources. Vitamin C is found in citrus fruits, tomatoes, strawberries, melon, green peppers, potatoes, and dark green vegetables. This is one vitamin where megadoses can definitely be dangerous, because the excess ascorbic acid is excreted in the urine, and acid urine promotes the formation of kidney stones.

Vitamin C capsules are available in health-food stores in strengths of 250, 500, and 1,000 milligrams. I don't recommend taking supplements routinely, but if you want to take Vitamin C for its antioxidant and cholesterol-lowering properties, 500 milligrams a day should suffice.

VITAMIN E (ALPHA-TOCOPHEROL)

At its annual meeting in June 1947 the American Medical Association issued the following statement: "Vitamin E is of no value in coronary heart disease, hypertension or rheumatic heart disease." The reason for making this edict and the subsequent reversal of opinion make an interesting story. Vitamin E was discovered in 1923 and was given the chemical name *tocopherol,* which refers to its first known property of preventing degeneration of the reproductive organs and "assuring a normal birth." It gained fame in 1947, when a series of articles were published in a medical journal by two Canadian physicians, Drs. Evan and Wilfrid Shute, who ran the Shute Institute in London, Ontario, and who were the first to propose that megadoses of vitamins may be beneficial. They claimed that large doses of vitamin E were good for treating a wide variety of cardiovascular diseases, including congestive heart failure, angina, hypertension, and intermittent claudication (pain in the legs during exercise resulting from an occluded blood supply). The rationale for their treatment was an observation that cattle fed a vitamin E–free diet developed weakness of their hearts and dropped dead, and they also postulated that vitamin E was a vasodilator (or, in other words, that it opened up constricted vessels). No mention was made of the antioxidant property of vitamin E, which in fact was not discovered until 1962, and even then its significance was not appreciated. The Shutes' claims for the dramatic healing properties of vitamin E were based on the reports of patients who were given the vitamin and said that they felt better, and were subsequently reported in *The New York Times* and other newspapers. Other more skeptical investigators went on to perform controlled trials in patients with conditions such as angina and claudication, which produced uniformly negative results. Since the Shutes did not carry out controlled trials, the benefits that they observed were almost certainly attributable to the placebo effect. Undaunted by the evidence and the accusation of quackery by the medical establishment, they went on to publish a book called *Vitamin E for Ailing and Healthy Hearts* in 1969.

Vitamin E gradually fell into disrepute, and when Dr. Robert Olson reviewed the situation in the journal *Circulation* in 1973, he concluded that there was no evidence of any effectiveness for patients with cardiovascular disease.

In the subsequent 20 years the wheel has turned full circle, and people with heart disease are now being advised to take vitamin E once more. This has occurred because of the gradual recognition of the importance of oxidation in the development of atherosclerosis and mounting evidence from epidemiological studies that vitamin E may help to prevent heart disease. With the wisdom of hindsight, it now appears that the quacks were right (but for the wrong reason), while the academic physicians were wrong (but for the right reason).

Following the publication of two large-scale trials in the *New England Journal of Medicine* in May 1993, both showing that people who consumed vitamin E are at lower risk of developing coronary heart disease, vitamin E became so much in demand that the health-food stores ran out of supplies. Why all the fuss? Vitamin E is an antioxidant and, as discussed above, is thought to inhibit the formation of atheroma.

The first of the two studies was the Nurses' Health Study, in which 87,245 nurses completed an extensive diet questionnaire, which included an evaluation of vitamin E intake, and were then followed for up to 8 years. The second, similar in design, was the Health Professionals Follow-Up Study, which was conducted in 39,000 male dentists, veterinarians, and the like, all of whom were followed for 4 years. Both studies came to the same conclusion, that taking vitamin E in a dose of 100 IU (international units) per day or more was associated with a nearly 50 percent reduction in the probability of developing coronary heart disease. Interestingly, neither study found any benefit from taking vitamin C, another antioxidant. The authors of both studies concluded that the results could not be explained away on the basis of the increased vitamin E intake being simply a marker for increased health consciousness (that is to say, that other health-related behaviors might have accounted for the benefits).

These two articles attracted an enormous amount of publicity, making the front page of major newspapers and the TV evening news, and hence the rush on vitamin E. At the same time the experts who conducted the study would not commit themselves to recommending that everybody should start taking vitamin E. Their argument was twofold: First, no controlled clinical trials have been conducted in which one group randomly allocated to take vitamin E is compared with a control group that does not. If the control group developed more heart disease, this would be definitive proof that the vitamin E was responsible. The second unresolved issue is the long-term effects of large doses, which are quite unknown. Nevertheless, it is worth noting that Dr. Stampfer, the first author of one of the *New England Journal* articles, and a coauthor of the other, admitted at a press conference that he takes it himself.

The vitamin E story underwent a further convolution in 1994 (described by the press as The Great Vitamin Scare of 1994), when the results of a large-scale controlled clinical trial were published, which at first sight appeared to contradict the earlier findings. This was a study of 29,000 Finnish men, all of whom were smokers. They were divided into four groups, one of which took vitamin E, one beta-carotene, one both, and one placebo (inert treatment). Over the next five years, there was no evidence for any protective effect of either of the two antioxidants on either heart disease or cancer. There was even a slight increase in the number of deaths from cerebral hemorrhage in the men given vitamin E, which resulted in the news media reporting the study as showing that vitamin E is harmful. Even worse, the incidence of lung cancer was 18 percent higher in the men who took beta-carotene than in those who didn't. The explanation for the lack of benefit from vitamin E is straight-forward: the dose used was only 50 IU per day, which is smaller than the dose used in the studies that did show benefit from vitamin E (100–400 IU).

There is no known disease associated with deficiency of vitamin E, but experiments done in animals have shown that its absence can cause damage to the heart and arteries. Its importance is as an antioxidant, and it has been shown to be able to prevent experimental atherosclerosis in rabbits. In humans, relatively small doses of vitamin E (200 IU a day) make blood platelets less sticky, an effect that should in theory resemble the benefits conferred by aspirin. In somewhat larger doses (1,200 IU a day), vitamin E may help to prevent the recurrence of blockage of coronary arteries that have been opened up by balloon angioplasty, although so far this effect appears to be marginal. Vitamin E does not affect blood lipid levels.

In a survey of nearly 2,000 men in 16 European populations, Dr. Fred Gey and his colleagues found a strong negative relationship between blood levels of vitamin E and the mortality from coronary heart disease, such that men with the highest blood levels had the lowest death rates. They also made the startling observation that in 12 of the populations, the relationship with heart disease was closer for vitamin E levels than for blood pressure or cholesterol. High blood levels of vitamins A and C also contributed to low death rates.

Sources. Vitamin E is found in vegetable oils (particularly olive oil), margarine, wheat germ, whole-grain cereals and bread, dried beans, and green leafy vegetables.

Vitamin E capsules are available in health-food stores in strengths of 100, 400, and 1,000 IU. There are no known ill effects from taking megadoses. The generally recommended dose is 400 IU per day.

NIACIN (VITAMIN B$_3$, NICOTINIC ACID)

Niacin is also known as nicotinic acid and vitamin B$_3$; it is important to distinguish it from nicotinamide, which does not have the same benefi-cial effects.

This was the first vitamin for which there was evidence that taking doses larger than the RDA could benefit people with coronary heart disease. It does all the right things with blood lipids: it lowers total cholesterol, raises HDL cholesterol, and lowers triglycerides. In large doses (3 grams per day) it also reduces lipoprotein a, another risk factor for coronary heart disease.

Its benefits were very clearly established by one of the earliest large-scale clinical trials of the prevention of heart attacks, the Coronary Drug Project. In this study, 1,119 men who had survived one heart attack were treated with niacin, and compared with 2,789 who had also had a heart attack, and who were given placebo. After six years, the cholesterols of the niacin-treated group were 10 percent lower than in the control group; and after nine years the mortality was 11 percent lower. In three other studies, in all of which niacin was given in combination with another lipid-lowering agent, it has been shown either to reduce mortality or to retard the progression of atheromatous plaques.

Niacin comes in two forms: the regular short-acting preparation, which has to be taken three times a day, and slow-release preparations, which need be taken only once a day. The biggest problem with niacin is its side effects, of which the most prominent are flushing and itching in the face. This can largely be overcome by using only the slow- or time-release preparations and by building up the dose gradually to the therapeutic level (2,000 to 3,000 milligrams or 2 to 3 grams a day). An aspirin a day also helps to reduce the flushing. Other side effects include abnormal liver function tests, increased uric acid (the cause of gout), increased blood sugar (which means that diabetics should not take it), and stomach ulcers. A more palatable form of niacin is the time-release preparation, which causes less flushing. It has one major drawback, however, and that is that it appears to be more likely to cause liver damage than the regular preparation. This risk is small, particularly if the total dose is kept below 2 grams a day. It is also a good idea to have regular blood tests to check the effects of niacin on liver function as well as on lipids.

The best form of the slow-release preparations of niacin is probably one called Endur-acin, which contains the niacin in a wax matrix, and is better absorbed from the stomach than some of the other preparations. In a study performed in 200 subjects it was found that a dose of 1,500 milligrams per day lowered the cholesterol/HDL ratio by about 20 percent. Endur-acin appears to cause less side effects such as flushing and abnormal liver function tests than the other types of niacin. I now recommend the Endur-acin preparation routinely for my patients who would benefit from niacin. The usual dose is 1,500 milligrams per day.

Sources. Niacin is found in some foods that are themselves not good for heart disease, such as liver, meat, and eggs, but it also occurs in whole-grain cereals, nuts, and dried peas and beans.

BETA-CAROTENE

This chemical gets its name from carrots, which are one of its main sources. It is converted to vitamin A (retinol) in the body, but it may also be important in its own right, because it is itself an antioxidant, and has the capacity to protect cell membranes from damage by oxidants. Low levels of beta-carotene in the blood have been consistently associated with lung cancer, and there is also evidence from several population surveys that people who eat a lot of vegetables and fruits are at lower risk of developing cancer of the lung and other sites. This does not necessarily mean that it is the beta-carotene which is giving the protection, however, for it is only one of more than 500 related substances called carotenoids present in vegetables, many of which may be more effective as antioxidants than beta-carotene.

Whether it's worth taking beta-carotene supplements is very questionable at the present time. The largest study to test its benefit was the one done on 29,000 Finnish male smokers (described in the section on vitamin E above), which found not only no evidence of any protective effect against cancer or heart disease, but an 8 percent higher mortality in the group taking beta-carotene, which was statistically significant (i.e., not due to chance). I would not recommend taking it, therefore.

Sources. Beta-carotene is found in carrots, green vegetables, squash, melon, and tomatoes.

FOLIC ACID

This vitamin got its name because it was originally extracted from spinach leaves, and was found to be effective in preventing certain types of anemia. It's found in other sorts of leafy vegetables and in orange juice, and the recommended daily intake is 200 micrograms.

Its importance in preventing heart disease is only just beginning to be accepted. It helps to keep down the levels of homocysteine (see Chapter 4), an amino acid that is normally present in the blood, but which in excessive amounts can damage the linings of arteries and lead to atherosclerosis. Vitamins B_6 and B_{12} also help to remove homocysteine. Folic acid deficiency is one of the most common types of vitamin deficiency, and it has been estimated that as many as 40 percent of Americans do not get enough folic acid to keep their homocysteine levels low.

Sources. Folic acid is available as a nonprescription medication in a dose of 0.4 milligram (400 mcg) in products such as One-A-Day and Theragran Stress Formula. It can also be obtained as a prescription medicine in larger doses. There are no known toxic effects from taking large amounts of folic acid, but in people who are deficient in vitamin B_{12} (a condition called pernicious anemia) it can mask the damaging effects of the B_{12} deficiency on the nerves. This is the reason why large doses are available only on prescription.

WHAT SHOULD I DO—TAKE VITAMINS OR EAT VEGETABLES?

On July 1, 1992, the National Cancer Institute gave a press conference for fruits and vegetables, an unusual topic for such hoopla. Its purpose was to announce its "Five a Day" Program, which was the suggestion that people should eat at least five, and as many as nine, half-cup servings of fruits and vegetables every day, on the grounds that this may reduce the risks of cancer and atherosclerotic heart disease. Since, as we have seen above, there is impressive evidence that many of the beneficial effects of this type of diet are likely to derive from vitamins, particularly the antioxidants, the manufacturers of vitamins, which include corporate giants such as Hoffman LaRoche, BASF Fine Chemicals, and General Nutrition Products, have been aggressively marketing their products. At a New York Academy of Sciences conference in February 1992, which was partly funded by Hoffman LaRoche, press releases made claims such as: "Vitamins found to offer major protective benefits" and "Antioxidant vitamins can slow some effects of aging."

If we all ate a balanced diet and followed the recommendations of the National Cancer Institute, you might argue that there would be no need to take any vitamin supplements. Most of us do not eat a balanced diet, however, and the experts are agreed that popping vitamins is no substitute for changing diets. As Regina Ziegler (a nutritional epidemiologist at the National Cancer Institute) said:

Our evidence implicates a protective role for fruits and vegetables some-what more clearly than the role for micronutrients. We want people to fo-cus more on fruits and vegetables. We aren't sure which ones, so we want them to eat a variety. It may also be prudent to take a one-a-day vitamin. What is dumb is to ignore your diet and what also is dumb is megadoses of vitamins, which interfere with absorption of other nutrients.

I would agree with this statement, with the only proviso that I believe that there is now sufficient evidence that large doses (for example, 400 IU per day) of vitamin E are protective against heart disease. Since it is difficult if not impossible to get this amount simply from eating vegeta-bles, I would advocate taking vitamin E.

WHICH BRANDS OF VITAMINS ARE BEST?

The numbers of available brands of vitamins are bewildering, and so is the range of prices. *Consumer Reports* published a good review of the market in the September 1994 edition. They pointed out that there is no control by the FDA or other regulatory agency of the manufacture and quality control of vitamins (although that could change in the near fu-ture). They tested 21 brands of vitamins C and E, and 18 of beta-carotene, and concluded that virtually all of them actually did contain what they were supposed to. The most striking finding was the range of prices: a bottle of 100 pills of 400 IU of vitamin E could cost as little as $3.76 (Spring Valley brand, sold by Wal-Mart) or as much as $16.65 (GNC Dry Natural). One explanation for this huge difference is that vitamin E is sold both as a "natural" and as a synthetic form. The nat-ural form costs about twice as much as the synthetic form, but is not necessarily any better, and all pills with 400 IU have about the same potency. So if you're going to take vitamin supplements, it pays to shop around. Other cheap brands of vitamin E are AARP Pharmacy Service Formula 419 Econo-E ($4.39 per 100), Kroger ($4.58 per 100), LaVerdiere ($4.69 per 100), Osco ($4.99 per 100), and Walgreen's ($4.99 per 100).

HEALTH FOODS AND HERBAL REMEDIES

I have included health foods and herbal remedies in the same chapter as vitamins because they tend to be packaged in the same way and sold in the same stores. There the similarity stops, however. Vitamins are a well-defined group of chemicals with proven value, at any rate in small doses, while the other health foods include many that are not only of no benefit but in some cases potentially harmful.

I have no problem in accepting that herbal remedies may be effective, because there are numerous examples in the history of medicine where such remedies have led to the identification of the active ingredient, which has then been incorporated into mainstream medicine. Aspirin is perhaps the best-known example, but others are digitalis (used for treating heart failure) and reserpine (the first effective blood-pressure-lowering drug, which was isolated from an Indian root used in folk medicine). We should also recognize, however, that while there may be many as yet undiscovered therapeutically active ingredients in herbal remedies, these same ingredients could have as many undesirable as desirable effects. A herbal remedy is basically a drug wrapped up in a leaf, and just as there are good drugs and bad drugs, so are there good herbs and bad herbs. There is a small but increasing number of reports in the medical literature of people being poisoned by consuming large amounts of some herbal teas.

I would also caution against the uncritical acceptance of remedies that are labeled as being "natural," which many people equate with non-toxic. The hemlock that killed Socrates was "natural," and coumadin, the blood thinner that is also used as rat poison, was originally extracted from clover. So be cautious.

Garlic

Garlic is one of the oldest medicines known. The Egyptians gave it to their slaves to increase their health and endurance; the Greek physician Hippocrates prescribed it for infections, cancer, and leprosy, and the medieval Europeans used it to ward off evil spirits. It is a member of the onion family of plants, and garlic and onions have similar therapeutic effects. Garlic may be more potent, but most of us would rather eat large amounts of onions than of garlic. I have classified garlic as a health food rather than a dietary component since when it is consumed for health reasons it is usually taken as pills bought in a health-food store rather than as food bought in a supermarket.

Despite its long medicinal history, garlic has been largely ignored by the medical profession. A recent analysis of the results of studies using garlic, published in the *Journal of the Royal College of Physicians of*

London by Drs. Christopher Silagy and Andrew Neil, concluded that it is beneficial, however. The active ingredient of garlic is an oil called allicin, whose most important therapeutic effect is to lower cholesterol. Drs. Silagy and Neil pooled the results of 16 trials of garlic conducted in nearly 1,000 patients, and concluded that there was an overall reduction in total cholesterol of 12 percent with a daily dose of 600 to 900 milligrams (a dose approximately equivalent to one medium-sized clove of fresh garlic). A similar fall in triglycerides was reported, but no change in HDL cholesterol. Some of the studies used a preparation of garlic powder called Kwai (taken as six capsules a day); in one the patients were hypertensive, and the garlic pills lowered the systolic blood pressure by 11 mm Hg. There were apparently no serious side effects, although some of the patients did report a noticeable smell of garlic.

While these results are encouraging, the number of patients who have been studied is still quite small, and six capsules a day are a lot to swallow.

Sources. There is a limit to how many cloves of garlic most of us can eat, but it is available as pills containing 300 or 1,000 milligrams. Kwai pills (see above) can also be obtained in the United States.

LECITHIN

This is an extract of soybeans that is alleged to lower blood cholesterol and to improve memory. If it does lower cholesterol at all, it is only because it is a polyunsaturated fat. Otherwise there is nothing special about it. There is no evidence that it improves memory.

NATURAL DIURETICS

If you shop in health-food stores you may come across pills that are claimed to be "natural" diuretics. An example is Nature's Bounty Water Pill, which contains buchu leaves, uva-ursi leaves, parsley leaves, juniper berries, and potassium gluconate. Buchu is a South African shrub that has been used as a herbal remedy for more than 200 years, and was first introduced to the United States in 1847 by a patent medicine entrepreneur named Henry Hembold, as Hembold's Compound Extract of Buchu for urinary problems, kidney stones, and "diseases arising from imprudence," the latter being a Victorian euphemism for venereal disease. Hembold made his fortune from this, and called himself the Buchu King.

Uva-ursi is related to cranberries, and from 1820 to 1936 was included in the U.S. Pharmacopoeia as a urinary antiseptic.

Juniper was advocated as a diuretic by the seventeenth-century English herbalist Nicholas Culpeper, but it has been reported to cause kidney damage in large doses.

I am unaware of any scientific studies of the efficacy of these agents, and do not recommend them.

SUMMARY

• There's no need to take large doses of multiple vitamins, but 400 IU of vitamin E per day is a good idea.

• If your cholesterol is high, niacin (at least 1,000 mg per day) should help to keep it down. The slow-release forms are easier to take, but may cause liver changes.

• Garlic may also help your cholesterol and blood pressure a little, but you need to take a lot of pills.

CHAPTER TWENTY-FIVE

OVER-THE-COUNTER MEDICATIONS

At the end of the past century, Sir William Osler, one of the most distinguished physicians of his time, wrote:

> Man has an inborn craving for medicine. Heroic dosing for several generations has given his tissues a thirst for drugs. The desire to take medicine is one feature which distinguishes man, the animal, from his fellow creatures.

We are bombarded daily by television commercials exhorting us to take pills and potions for the relief of headaches, colds, flu, heartburn, acid indigestion, and constipation. In this chapter I will review some of the more commonly used over-the-counter medications, and whether they are safe or desirable to take if you have high blood pressure.

ASPIRIN: THE AGELESS PANACEA

In 1763 the Reverend Edward Stone of Chipping Norton, a peaceful village in the Cotswolds of England, wrote a letter to the Royal Society, the country's most prestigious scientific organization, describing his discovery of the benefit of willow bark for relieving the pains of arthritis. He concluded his letter as follows: "I have no other motives for publishing this valuable specific than that it may have a fair and full trial that the world may reap the benefits accruing from it." Today, more than 200 years later, his wish has been more than fulfilled, and almost every year sees the discovery of new benefits of taking aspirin. The active ingredient of willow bark is salicylic acid, and aspirin, whose chemical name is acetylsalicylate, is a more palatable derivative of it. Aspirin is now the most widely used medication in the world, and in the United States alone over 15,000 tons of it are manufactured every year. That's an awful lot of pills.

HOW ASPIRIN WORKS

The mechanism by which aspirin exerts its effect is by blocking the formation of a family of chemicals called prostaglandins. These have a wide variety of actions in the body, one of the most important of which is the promotion of inflammation, the swelling of tissues that occurs in response to injury. This explains aspirin's pain-relieving effect. Prostaglandins are also involved in the response to injury of the endothelium, which is the thin film of cells lining the inner surface of blood vessels. When the endothelium is injured, as for example by atherosclerosis, minute cells called blood platelets aggregate to form a plug over the damaged area. While this is clearly beneficial when the vessel is injured by mechanical trauma, it may lead to an occlusion or thrombosis of the vessel when it is injured by atherosclerosis. Again by blocking the formation of prostaglandins, aspirin makes the platelets less sticky. This explains both its most important beneficial effect—the prevention of thrombosis—and its most important side effect—bleeding.

AN ASPIRIN A DAY KEEPS THE DOCTOR AWAY

The benefits of aspirin for preventing heart disease have been most clearly established by the Physicians' Health Study. Twenty-two thousand male U.S. physicians, aged between 40 and 84, volunteered to take part in the study, and were randomly allocated to take either regular aspirin (325 mg of the coated form) or a placebo pill every other day. All were in good health at the start of the study, and after five years approximately half as many doctors in the aspirin group had suffered a heart attack as in the placebo group. There was no reduction in the number of strokes as a result of taking aspirin, and there was even a slight excess of strokes from cerebral hemorrhage, although this could have been a chance finding. There was no difference in overall mortality between the two groups. The doctors who took aspirin also reported more bleeding problems.

In people who have already suffered from the consequences of atherosclerotic disease, as either a stroke, a heart attack, or angina, the benefits are even more clear. Several randomized trials have been completed, and in patients who have already had strokes (from a thrombosis, but not from a hemorrhage) or ministrokes (also known as transient ischemic attacks or TIAs) aspirin reduces the risk of a subsequent stroke or heart attack by 20 percent.

HOW MUCH ASPIRIN IS NEEDED?

The early trials of aspirin used doses of 300 to 900 milligrams per day (1–3 regular aspirin pills), but there are theoretical reasons for thinking that smaller doses may have a greater protective effect. Blood platelets make two main types of prostaglandin: thromboxane and prostacyclin. Thromboxane makes platelets more sticky and constricts blood vessels, while prostacyclin does just the opposite. It has recently been discovered that much lower doses of aspirin may block the synthesis of thromboxane, while leaving the formation of prostacyclin intact. Although the data are not yet conclusive, there are now several studies, including one from Holland and another from Sweden, that suggest that a baby aspirin (containing 81 milligrams) may be just as effective as a regular one, and with reduced side effects.

SHOULD PEOPLE WITH HIGH BLOOD PRESSURE TAKE ASPIRIN?

None of the studies that have demonstrated the protective effect of aspirin was designed to test its effectiveness in people with high blood pressure. In the Physicians' Health Study, only 5 percent of subjects were hypertensive, although in some of the other studies up to 40 percent were. Since high blood pressure is a major risk factor for strokes and heart attacks, it might seem prudent to recommend that hypertensive patients should take aspirin routinely. Two qualifications are appropriate, however. First, the Physicians' Health Study showed no evidence of any benefit in people below the age of 50, and second, aspirin may increase the risk of a hemorrhagic (bleeding) stroke, to which hypertensive patients are particularly susceptible. There has not been a study that specifically tests the benefits (or harm) of taking aspirin in hypertensive subjects.

I do not routinely recommend aspirin for my patients unless they are over 50, their blood pressure is well controlled, and they have other cardiovascular risk factors.

OTHER BENEFITS OF ASPIRIN

Cancer of the colon accounts for about 12 percent of all cancer deaths in the United States. A recent observational study of more than 600,000 people published in the prestigious *New England Journal of Medicine* reported that those who took aspirin on a regular basis were at half the risk of developing cancer of the colon compared with those who did not. Two previous studies had found similar results. An editorial accompanying this report concluded that, while these findings are encouraging, it would be premature to recommend routine use of aspirin for cancer prevention. Nevertheless, this has the prospect of being another benefit of aspirin.

ADVIL AND OTHER NSAIDs

You have undoubtedly heard of Advil, but may be unclear as to what NSAID means. The acronym stands for nonsteroidal antiinflammatory drug (steroids being the other major class of drugs that suppress inflammation). Aspirin is one of them, but there are many others, two of which (ibuprofen and naproxen; see Table 25.1 for their brand names) are available without prescriptions. NSAIDs are the most commonly prescribed drugs worldwide, accounting for about 6 percent of all prescriptions. Their main use is for the treatment of arthritis, so they are used particularly often in the elderly.

A significant problem with NSAIDs is that they raise blood pressure. A recent review of 38 controlled trials concluded that the average increase was about 5 mm Hg, a sizable change. They didn't all have the same effect, however. For aspirin the effect was negligible. Sulindac and flurbiprofen also caused relatively little increase, while bigger changes were seen with indomethacin and ibuprofen. NSAIDs also tend to antagonize the effects of blood-pressure-lowering medication. Like aspirin, they can also cause stomach ulcers.

What this means in practice is that if you have high or borderline blood pressure and you take NSAIDs for any length of time, you should get your pressure checked.

Table 25.1. Generic and Brand Names of NSAIDs

GENERIC NAME	BRAND NAMES
Aspirin	Ecotrin, Ascriptin, Disalcid, Trisilate
Diclofenac sodium	Cataflam, Voltaren
Etodolac	Lodine
Fenoprofen calcium	Nalfon
Flurbiprofen	Ansaid
Ibuprofen	Advil, Motrin, Nuprin
Indomethacin	Indocin
Ketoprofen	Orudis
Naproxen	Naprosyn, Anaprox
Oxaprozin	Daypro
Piroxicam	Feldene
Sulindac	Clinoril
Tolmetin sodium	Tolectin

COUGH AND COLD REMEDIES

As a nation, we spend more than $1 billion a year on medicines for coughs, colds, and flu, despite the fact that none of them has any curative effect on the underlying disease, which is caused by a virus. As you will appreciate when you try to choose one in a drugstore, the number of brands available is quite bewildering. *The Physicians' Desk Reference* lists 437 different varieties of tablets, caplets, gelcaps, extentabs, chewables, powders, liqui-gels, elixirs, syrups, nighttime drinks, rubs, and sprays, all designed to rid us of "sinus colds' miseries."

The symptoms arise from dilation of the blood vessels of the mucosal membranes of the nose and throat, which causes the secretion of phlegm and the feeling of congestion. The medications are supposed to provide symptomatic relief, and they do this with varying mixtures of two main ingredients. The first is a vasoconstrictor, which is usually a derivative of the hormone norepinephrine. The ones most commonly used are ephedrine, pseudoephedrine, phenylephrine, and phenyl-propanolamine. While this vasoconstriction in the nose may help to relieve the symptoms, if it occurs elsewhere in the body it will, at any rate in theory, tend to raise the blood pressure. This is the reason why decongestants are generally not recommended for people with high blood pressure. In practice, however, this is not a significant problem. Studies in which decongestants such as phenylpropanolamine have been given every day for several weeks have not shown any consistent effect on blood pressure.

The other major ingredient is an antihistamine. This is most effective when the underlying problem is an allergic reaction such as hay fever or allergic rhinitis, and it is not of much help for a common cold. It has no tendency to raise the blood pressure, however, and the main side effect is to make you feel sleepy. Examples of antihistamines are brompheniramine and chlorpheniramine. Other ingredients may include analgesics (aspirin, acetaminophen, and ibuprofen) and cough suppressants (dextromethorphan), none of which poses any particular problems for people with high blood pressure.

To find out which medicines contain the vasoconstrictors, you need to look at the small print on the packet. Going by the brand name is not enough: Dristan comes in 16 different formulations, and as shown in Table 25.2, their composition varies greatly.

Table 25.2. Composition of Different Varieties of Dristan

	DRISTAN JUICE MIX-IN PACKET	MAXIMUM STRENGTH DRISTAN GEL CAPLET	MAXIMUM STRENGTH DRISTAN COATED CAPLET	DRISTAN COLD COATED TABLET	DRISTAN ALLERGY COATED CAPLET	DRISTAN SINUS COATED CAPLET
Analgesics						
Acetaminophen	500	500	500	325	—	—
Ibuprofen	—	—	—	—	—	200
Decongestants						
Pseudoephedrine	60	30	30	—	60	30
Phenylephrine	—	—	—	5	—	—
Antihistamines						
Brompheniramine	—	2	—	—	4	—
Chlorpheniramine maleate	—	—	—	2	—	—
Cough suppressant						
Dextromethorphan	20	—	—	—	—	—

Source: *Physicians' Desk Reference*. Doses are in milligrams.

The advice I usually give my patients about using these medicines is that if your blood pressure is well controlled, and you're taking them for only a short period of time in the recommended doses, there should be no problem.

SUMMARY

• There's no need to take aspirin routinely if you have high blood pressure unless you have multiple other risk factors, or are known to have vascular disease.

• Nonsteroidal analgesics (NSAIDs) can raise blood pressure and cause stomach ulcers, so take them sparingly.

• You can take cough and cold remedies, which have a negligible effect on blood pressure.

CHAPTER TWENTY-SIX

PSYCHOLOGICAL METHODS OF TREATMENT

There is absolutely no doubt that being aroused raises your blood pressure. In our own research we have found that most people's pressure is highest when they are at work, and drops by 5 mm Hg or more when they go home in the evening. And when they're watching television it's lowest of all, except for sleep. So if stress and mental tension play any role in the development of hypertension (a view that is not accepted by many physicians; see Chapter 8), you might suppose that reduction of stress and the use of relaxation modes should help to control it. A whole host of techniques for doing this has been developed, such as biofeedback, meditation, yoga, autogenic training, and progressive muscular relaxation. Despite their different-sounding names, they are in fact very similar. They all have two crucial features—muscular relaxation and the focusing of attention, both of which will tend to lower blood pressure. The general idea underlying the use of such techniques is that if they are practiced on a continuing and regular basis they will lead to a sustained reduction in blood pressure—a leap of faith that may or may not be justified.

The general approach has been around for a long time, but really came into vogue in the 1970s, principally due to the work of two men, Dr. Herbert Benson, who introduced the "relaxation response," and Dr. Neal Miller, whose research provided the origins of biofeedback. In the next ten years there was a flurry of activity by clinical psychologists, and many extravagant claims were made for the number of diseases that could be successfully treated using these new drug-free methods, ranging from epilepsy to diabetes, and including, of course, high blood pressure. I well remember the air of excitement at one of the early meetings of the Biofeedback Society of America in 1972, when a psychologist stated that it was now possible, after only a few training sessions, to "learn to drive your own body."

These early expectations were not fulfilled, however, and today these techniques have not found wide acceptance among the medical profession.

BIOFEEDBACK

The technique of biofeedback originated in Dr. Neal Miller's research into what he called "visceral learning." The nervous system has traditionally been divided into two components—the voluntary and the involuntary, or autonomic, nervous system. The former regulates the activity of the skeletal muscles, and is under our conscious control. The latter regulates the activity of the heart and "smooth" muscle, and is controlled by the brain subconsciously. Dr. Miller's revolutionary idea was that the reason we are normally unable to constrict and dilate our blood vessels voluntarily is that we are unable to sense what their state of contraction is. He argued that if this information was provided (as "biofeedback"), we might be able to regulate our bodily functions voluntarily. Thus, if you want people to learn how to lower their blood pressure, you could hook them up to a monitor that sounds a tone whenever the blood pressure goes down. You then ask them to try to keep the tone sounding as much as possible. Another method uses a more indirect approach and provides feedback from the forehead (or other) muscles, on the grounds that relaxing these muscles lowers the blood pressure. You don't need to know exactly how you're keeping your pressure down in order to be able to learn this skill.

RELAXATION TRAINING

The concept of the "relaxation response" was first developed by Dr. Herbert Benson, and is regarded as being the mirror image of the "fight-or-flight" response. It is characterized by bodily relaxation and a reduction in heart rate and blood pressure and also in oxygen consumption. In some ways these are the same changes that occur during sleep, although in this case consciousness is maintained. The idea is not a new one, and has been incorporated into the practice of several religions; Dr. Benson has traced it back to the fourteenth century in Christianity and even further in Eastern religions. During the practice of yoga, Zen, and transcendental meditation, the same changes occur. A common feature of all these procedures is the repetition of a single word, which is aimed to block out thoughts of worldly things.

Dr. Benson's instructions are to sit quietly in a comfortable position, close your eyes, relax your muscles, and repeat a word such as "one" with each breath. He recommends practicing it for 10 to 20 minutes twice a day.

AUTOGENIC TRAINING AND PROGRESSIVE MUSCULAR RELAXATION

These two procedures are generally similar to relaxation training, except that the attention is more directly focused on relaxing specific muscle groups.

HOW EFFECTIVE ARE THESE PROCEDURES AT LOWERING BLOOD PRESSURE?

Although there have been a large number of widely publicized studies claiming that these techniques can produce significant reductions in blood pressure, there are others, less well publicized, that have found them to be relatively ineffective. No one technique emerges as clearly superior to any other. Some researchers have found that the blood pressure reductions following biofeedback, relaxation training, or both are no greater than those seen after simply giving patients instructions to relax, or even giving no instructions at all.

The biggest problem with these procedures, however, is that there is little or no evidence that their blood-pressure-lowering effects are sustained. Relaxation training may indeed be very effective at lowering your pressure while you are consciously relaxing, but there is no good reason to suppose that doing this for 20 minutes twice a day should result in any sustained reduction of pressure throughout the day and night. In fact, what few studies have been done using ambulatory monitoring have mostly shown no reduction following treatment with these procedures. This brings us to the question of whether the reported changes can be regarded as a placebo effect.

THE PLACEBO EFFECT: IT'S ALL IN THE MIND

The Latin word *placebo* means "I will please," and the placebo effect occurs when a treatment is therapeutically inert but makes the patient feel better. This improvement is usually only subjective, but may include objective changes, of which an apparent reduction in blood pressure is one example. With a few notable exceptions, it is only in the last 60 years or so that doctors have had drugs that actually do anything useful, and yet doctors have enjoyed prestige for much longer than that, largely thanks to the placebo effect. Before the introduction of the first really effective antihypertensive medication in 1951, numerous remedies for hypertension (such as extract of watermelon seed) had been advocated, some of them with surprising success.

In 1956 Dr. William Goldring and his colleagues designed an ingenious experiment to investigate the effectiveness of reassurance and the placebo effect in hypertensive patients. They made an impressive-looking device that they called an "electron gun," which consisted of a large metal coil surmounted by a conical "gun" and an oscilloscope. The patient was seated in a darkened room, with the gun pointing at his or her chest. When it was turned on, the nozzle of the gun began to glow as if it were red hot and to emit sparks and crackling sounds. At the same time a series of sinusoidal waves was displayed on the oscilloscope.

The treatment was carried out by a sympathetic nurse twice a week for several months, and then discontinued. In about half of the patients the blood pressure decreased during the treatment period, with an average drop of 36/27 (systolic/diastolic) mm Hg—a very impressive change. In addition, the patients all reported an improvement in their symptoms, and several were able to return to work. However, once the treatment was discontinued, the pressure gradually climbed back to pretreatment levels.

How should these results be interpreted? Was this a real improvement in these patients' blood pressure? The simplest explanation is that the psychological reassurance that this treatment provided resulted in a dampening of the increase in blood pressure that occurred when the patients went to the clinic (we have termed this increase the white-coat effect, and discuss it in more detail in Chapter 10), without having any sustained effect on the blood pressure at other times. But then, you might say, why did the symptoms get better, if the fall of blood pressure was so transient? The answer is that the symptoms were not directly due to the high blood pressure, but to the associated anxiety. As the authors concluded, "We have no reason to suspect that the observed reduction in pressure reflects any alteration in the basic and unknown process or processes underlying the hypertensive state." They did not recommend using the electron gun in clinical practice.

When I visited the Soviet Union in 1982 as a member of a scientific delegation, one of our more memorable experiences was being taken to a sanitarium set in pine woods on the Baltic coast, and being shown the treatments that were being used for a variety of diseases. A device very similar to the electron gun, which was placed over the patient's head, was used to treat migraine. For other conditions there were other devices—pressurization chambers, suction chambers, and laser beam acupuncture machines. All of them had one feature in common: they looked (and in some cases sounded) very impressive and, so far as we skeptical Westerners were aware, had absolutely no scientific basis for their use. I am equally sure, however, that the patients' symptoms improved, in just the same way as Dr. Goldring's patients' did.

An interesting analysis of the nonspecific effects in healing was carried out by Dr. Alan Roberts and his colleagues from the San Diego State University. They selected five forms of medical and surgical treatment that had once been considered to be efficacious by their proponents, but had in subsequent controlled trials been found to have no specific value and were later abandoned. One of the more colorful examples was freezing the stomach for treating stomach ulcers. This was accomplished by passing a stomach-shaped balloon through the patient's mouth and into the stomach, and then filling the balloon with cold absolute alcohol and leaving it for an hour. Its proponent was a well-known surgeon named Dr. Owen H. Wangensteen, who believed that it worked by killing off the cells in the stomach that make acid (and hence cause ulcers), and he referred to it as a "physiological gastrectomy." He published a series of enthusiastic reports in the 1960s, in which 98 to 100 percent of patients reported relief of their symptoms. Later studies conducted by other more skeptical surgeons, which included control groups who did not get their stomachs frozen, found that the treatment groups did no better than the controls, and the procedure fell into disfavor. One suspects that one reason Dr. Wangensteen's patients reported such good results was their fear that if they admitted that their symptoms were coming back, Dr. Wangensteen would get out his balloon once more.

The overall results of the five procedures reviewed by Dr. Roberts were remarkably consistent: 40 percent of patients had excellent results, 30 percent good, and 30 percent reported little or no improvement. The important conclusion reached by Dr. Roberts and his colleagues was that if both the practitioner and the patient have high expectations that the treatment will make the patient feel better, it will in about 70 percent of cases, no matter what type of treatment is used. This, I believe, is the basis of the placebo response, and explains most of the apparent successes of "alternative" forms of medicine described in Chapter 27, as well as many of the successes of behavioral forms of treatment described in this one.

ARE THE RESULTS WITH BIOFEEDBACK AND RELAXATION DUE TO THE PLACEBO EFFECT?

Biofeedback and the other psychological treatment modalities share many of the features of the electron gun treatment. With biofeedback there is again the impressive electronic equipment, but more important is the establishment of contact with a sympathetic therapist, and a treatment that involves multiple visits over a prolonged period of time, all of which are features that should foster the placebo effect. Furthermore, studies comparing the efficacy of the different modes of behavioral treatment have not shown any superiority of one modality over another, which would also be consistent with the effects being nonspecific. And finally, evidence that these forms of treatment can produce a sustained lowering of blood pressure throughout the day and night is lacking.

I advise my patients that if they are tense and anxious, these treatments may help them feel better, but they should not have high expectations that their blood pressure will show much improvement.

SUMMARY

• Biofeedback and relaxation training may make you feel better, but they're unlikely to have much effect on your blood pressure.

• Many of the reported benefits of this type of treatment are placebo effects.

CHAPTER TWENTY-SEVEN

ALTERNATIVE MEDICINE

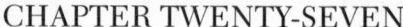

I use the term *alternative medicine* to describe a number of therapeutic procedures that are at or beyond the fringes of acceptability by the medical establishment. *Unconventional medicine* and *fringe medicine* are also commonly used descriptors. They have one common feature, which is the lack of any convincing scientific evidence that they work. It is certainly possible that some of them are genuinely effective and that the appropriate studies have simply not been carried out, but I am skeptical, and some, like chelation therapy, can be downright dangerous. Another feature that characterizes these treatments is that the physician or therapist prescribing them is also the person who will be billing you for them, and most of them require several sessions or dosings, so the practitioners of these arts have a direct financial interest in their promotion.

The alternative medicine business is doing very well. A recent survey found that 10 percent of Americans had consulted providers of unconventional forms of treatment in the past year, with an average of 19 visits at a cost of $27.60 per visit. In 1990 that all added up to an expenditure of $13.7 billion, most of which was paid out of pocket. This is a figure comparable to the amount spent out of pocket annually for all hospitalizations in the United States. High blood pressure was among the top 10 conditions for which people used alternative medicine, and most people did not consult their doctors or tell them they were doing so.

To some extent, the success of fringe medicine is a consequence of the failings of modern conventional medicine: as physicians we are becoming more and more reliant on technology for diagnosing and treating our patients, and we can make much more money by performing procedures than by talking or listening to our patients. In many cases people feel better as a result of using fringe medicine, and while I would voice the opinion that this is usually because of the placebo effect, I also believe that most physicians underestimate the importance of this.

Most forms of fringe medicine can be regarded as fraud or quackery. Its advocates often have little or no scientific qualifications, although a distressingly large number of them are M.D.s. They spread their messages of hope by writing books, appearing on television talk shows, and even having their own radio shows. Because there is so much money involved, the media welcome them with open arms. In fact, the more outrageous the claim, the more newsworthy is the claimant. In his book called *A Consumer's Guide to Alternative Medicine*, Kurt Butler describes how talk show hosts such as Phil Donahue, Oprah Winfrey, and Sally Jessy Raphael aid and abet these practitioners by inviting them to appear on their shows. Respectable book publishers have done very well by publishing flagrantly unreliable and inaccurate texts, which Butler describes as "health pornography."

The National Institutes of Health have now been mandated to investigate the scientific utility, or lack of it, of fringe medicine. In 1992 the Office of Alternative Medicine was set up to award research grants to investigators who were planning to test some of these techniques. One of the advocates of this development was Senator Tom Harkin, who chaired the Senate Appropriations Committee, and who believed that his allergies had been cured by the use of bee pollen.

Although there is no precise definition of alternative or fringe medicine, the techniques fall into two general categories. The first involves the use of chemicals or drugs, such as chelation therapy, homeopathy, and herbal remedies, and the second are the "mind-body" approaches such as spiritual healing, meditation, and acupuncture. I have discussed some of these elsewhere—for example, herbal remedies in Chapter 24, and meditation in Chapter 26.

In evaluating the usefulness of the variety of techniques of alternative medicine, we should keep an open mind, but be skeptical. Just because a practitioner of a particular mode of healing tells us that it works is no reason why we should believe him (or her), any more than we should believe a used-car salesman who tells us what an incredible bargain we're getting. Two general criteria by which to judge a form of treatment are, first, that it should be biologically plausible and, second, that there should be some objective evidence of success. Herbal remedies and chelation therapy are certainly plausible, since they both involve the administration of drugs or chemicals, albeit in an unconventional form. This does not guarantee that they are either safe or effective, however; there has never been a drug that is without undesirable side effects, and probably never will be. At the same time, I have a real problem in accepting homeopathy, which defies common sense because the drugs used may be so dilute that they are nonexistent.

Objective evidence of success is, almost by definition, lacking for alternative forms of medicine. If and when such evidence is obtained, it will cease to be "alternative" and will gain acceptance by mainstream physicians. Perhaps the best example of this is the vitamin E story, which I describe in Chapter 24. When I was a medical student, taking more than the recommended daily dose of vitamin E was regarded as quackery, but now I prescribe it for many of my patients.

CHELATION THERAPY

In 1992 a book was published entitled *Forty Something Forever: A Consumer's Guide to Chelation Therapy,* by Harold and Arline Brecher. According to the authors, whom the cover describes as being "Two crack medical journalists," this form of treatment will accomplish the following goals:

- Retard atherosclerosis
- Reduce high blood pressure
- Normalize weight
- Improve arthritis
- Reverse hair loss
- Reverse impotence
- Reverse symptoms of Alzheimer's disease
- Overcome chronic fatigue syndrome
- Reduce mortality from cancer by 90 percent
- Produce a more youthful appearance, including more lustrous hair, added eye sparkle, stronger unsplit nails, better skin color, and fewer visible wrinkles

All I can say is that, if you believe this, you will believe anything. I'll go farther and say that the chemistry of the body is so complex, and the innumerable disturbances that produce disease so subtle, that no single treatment will ever be able to help a range of diseases such as this.

Actually, there is nothing new about chelation therapy. Its basis is a chemical called EDTA (for ethylenediaminetetraacetic acid), which was first synthesized in 1935. The word *chelation* is derived from the Greek word for claw, and chelation agents grab certain chemicals, particularly metals, with which they come in contact. EDTA has an approved and well-substantiated use as treatment for lead poisoning, and it has also been advocated for exposure to radioactive fallout.

Its use as a treatment for atherosclerosis dates back to the 1950s, when workers in a battery factory were being treated with EDTA for lead poisoning. During this treatment, some of them reported that their angina pains improved.

Since that time "chelation clinics" have been established for the treatment of atherosclerosis and other disorders all over the country. The EDTA is given intravenously as a course of up to 10 treatments over a two- or three-month period. Despite its long history, and the extravagant claims for it, there has never been a properly controlled scientific study of its value in atherosclerosis. It also has serious side effects: it lowers the level of calcium in the blood, which can cause arrhythmias, respiratory arrest, and muscle spasms, and it can also cause serious kidney damage. The FDA has not received any applications by any of the many physicians using it to document its value, and the manufacturers of EDTA are so skeptical about it that they have not thought it worthwhile to sponsor such studies. There are now several published studies showing that drug treatment can promote the regression of atherosclerotic plaques, but not one of them has been done with EDTA. In a letter about chelation clinics to the medical journal *Chest* published in 1984, Dr. Alfred Soffer wrote that, having reviewed the published literature on the subject, he concluded that chelation therapy "does not significantly alter the course of coronary disease, nor does it offer any protection against repeated infarctions and death." And the Brechers titled one of the chapters in their book "What's New about EDTA Chelation? Nothing! That's Really Big News."

HOMEOPATHY—MUCH ADO ABOUT NOTHING

The principle of homeopathy, which was developed 200 years ago by the German physician Samuel Hahnemann, is that the administration of tiny doses of a drug that causes symptoms resembling the disease when given in larger doses to healthy people will help to cure the disease. He formulated the basic homeopathic law, that "like cures like," after experimenting with cinchona bark, which contains quinine and was known to cure malaria. After taking the drug, he experienced symptoms similar to those of malaria, including palpitations, flushing, and thirst. Following this experience he constructed an entire edifice of treatments for different disorders by matching the symptoms of the disorder with the side effects of the drugs. If, for example, you have kidney disease, your treatment will be a little arsenic, because larger amounts of arsenic cause kidney damage.

Scientifically, this doesn't make any sense, because the dilutions used are so extensive that there may not be a single molecule of the prescribed medication left by the time the patient takes it. Hahnemann tried to get around this problem by claiming that the vigorous shaking that is part of the dilution process somehow "potentizes" the solution. Again, this makes no sense. Despite this lack of any sound scientific basis, homeopathy continues to have many advocates, including the British royal family. A recent survey of 293 general physicians in Holland found that 45 percent of them thought that homeopathic remedies are effective in treating upper respiratory tract infections.

Whether there is any objective evidence that homeopathy has a genuine therapeutic effect was reviewed by Professor Paul Knipschild and his colleagues at the University of Limburg in Holland. They surveyed the medical literature and found 107 controlled trials of homeopathy in the treatment of a whole host of disorders, including hypertension. Although most of the studies were of poor quality scientifically, they concluded that the evidence was sufficiently encouraging to warrant further well-controlled studies. Only three studies examined the treatment of hypertension; two concluded that the treatment was ineffective. The third claimed positive results, but scored only 13 out of a possible maximum of 100 for scientific validity, so little credence can be placed on its conclusions.

ACUPUNCTURE

According to the U.S. Food and Drug Administration, approximately 10 million acupuncture treatments are performed every year in the United States, mostly for the control of pain and addictions. It is undoubtedly one of the oldest forms of medical treatment, having been around for at least 2,500 years, but there's still no conclusive scientific evidence that it's anything more than a placebo. It involves the insertion of needles into a variety of specific sites in the body, the locations of which depend on the condition being treated. However, the traditional Chinese concepts of disease are very different from our Western ideas. Good health is regarded as a balance between the opposing forces of yin and yang, and the attraction between them creates an energy or life force known as qi. This flows through the body in 14 major meridians or channels, and acupuncture aims to restore the balance of qi by inserting the needles at any of almost 200 locations along these channels.

CHIROPRACTIC

Most people think of chiropractic as a treatment for back pain, which of course it is, or claims to be. Chiropractors, however, also claim that it can be used to treat a variety of other conditions, including heart disease, asthma, and hypertension.

Chiropractic was founded by Daniel David Palmer, who had previously dabbled in magnetic healing, and established the Palmer School of Chiropractic in Davenport, Iowa, in 1895. It was expanded by his son B. J. Palmer, who was the first to award the school's graduates a Doctor of Chiropractic (D.C.) degree. Today there are several chiropractic colleges in the United States, chiropractors' qualifications are recognized in all 50 states, and their services are reimbursable through Medicare, Medicaid, and most major private insurance schemes.

You might be excused for thinking that this means that there is some scientific justification for the practice of chiropractic, but unfortunately this is not the case. The basic theory is that minor misalignments of the vertebrae (spine) interfere with the normal flow of "nerve energy" through the adjacent nerves, and hence cause malfunction of the organs they supply. How this can lead to such a variety of medical disorders is not specified, but in any event it doesn't matter, because whatever your problem, the treatment is the same—spinal manipulation.

Despite its veneer of respectability, this is one intervention that can be dangerous. Backs and necks have been broken and strokes have resulted from manipulations that have damaged the arteries in the neck.

SUMMARY

- Alternative medicine gets its name because its benefits, if any, are unproven and probably due to placebo effects.

- While some forms (e.g., homeopathy) are harmless, others such as chelation therapy and chiropractic can be dangerous. Avoid them.

GLOSSARY

Adrenaline. A hormone released by the adrenal glands that stimulates the heart and dilates the arteries. It is also referred to as epinephrine.

Aldosterone. A hormone released by the adrenal glands that acts on the kidney to retain salt and excrete potassium.

Alpha-adrenergic blocker. A drug that dilates arteries by blocking the constrictor effects of norepinephrine, and hence lowers blood pressure.

Alpha receptors. Regions on the walls of the muscle cells of arteries and veins to which norepinephrine can attach itself and cause the muscle to contract.

Aneroid. A type of sphygmomanometer that has a dial to register the pressure rather than a mercury column.

Aneurysm. A weak spot in the wall of an artery that balloons out and may eventually burst.

Angina pectoris. The Latin words for pain in the chest, which results from a shortage of oxygen in the heart muscle, usually because of a blockage in the arteries to the heart or more rarely because of spasm.

Angiogram. See Arteriogram.

Angiotensin blocking agents. A new class of drugs that act by blocking the actions of angiotensin. Also known as AT I antagonists.

Angiotensin converting enzyme (ACE) inhibitor. A drug that lowers blood pressure by blocking the formation of angiotensin, a substance that constricts arteries.

Ankle-arm index. The ratio of the blood pressure in the ankle to the pressure in the arm, which is normally 1. A ratio below 0.9 is an indicator of atherosclerotic disease.

Antioxidants. Substances that inhibit the actions of unstable forms of oxygen (free radicals), which can accelerate the development of atherosclerosis and cancer.

Aorta. The main artery of the body, into which blood is pumped from the heart. It arches over the heart and runs down through the chest into the abdomen, where it divides into two main branches going to the legs.

Arrhythmia. A disturbance of the normal and regular heart rhythm. There are several different types of arrhythmia; some are dangerous, most are not.

Arteries. The blood vessels that branch off the aorta, and carry oxygenated blood at high pressure to the tissues of the body,

Arteriogram or angiogram. An X ray of the arteries, taken after injecting dye (contrast medium) into the artery through a plastic cannula (tube).

Arterioles. The arteries divide into smaller and smaller branches, called arterioles, which have muscle in their walls and can actively contract and relax.

Arteriosclerosis or atherosclerosis. The process whereby cholesterol and other substances are deposited in the walls of the arteries, to form plaques that can eventually block off the flow of blood.

Atherectomy. A process whereby atheromatous plaque is reamed out of a coronary artery by a catheter.

Autonomic nervous system. The "involuntary nervous system," which regulates bodily functions such as the circulation and digestion. Its main subdivisions are the sympathetic and parasympathetic systems.

Beta blockers. Drugs that block some of the effects of epinephrine and norepinephrine on the circulation, and thus slow the heart rate and lower the blood pressure.

Beta receptors. Regions on the heart and blood vessels to which norepinephrine and epinephrine can attach and cause physiological changes.

Blood pressure. The pressure existing in the arteries.

Blood volume. The total amount of blood in the circulation.

Bruit. A whooshing sound audible through a stethoscope of blood flowing through an artery, usually because a narrowing in the artery has caused turbulent flow.

Calcium-channel blocker. A drug that blocks the entry of calcium into the muscle cells of the arterioles (small blood vessels), and hence stops them contracting.

Capillaries. The smallest blood vessels, which form a fine network permeating the tissues.

Cardiac output. The amount of blood pumped by the heart in one minute.

Cardiovascular. Refers to the heart (cardio) and blood vessels (vascular).

Catecholamines. The hormones epinephrine (adrenaline) and norepinephrine (noradrenaline), which are released by the sympathetic nervous system and tend to raise the blood pressure.

Cholesterol. A fatty substance circulating in the blood and present in the tissues that is synthesized in the body and also comes from the diet. In excess amounts it may be deposited in the arterial walls as atherosclerotic plaques. It circulates in two forms, HDL and LDL cholesterol.

Claudication. Pain in the leg muscles that starts during walking and is relieved by rest. It is caused by atherosclerotic narrowing of the arteries supplying the legs.

Coarctation of the aorta. A constriction of the aorta that is a rare cause of hypertension in children.

Collateral circulation. When a major artery becomes blocked, smaller (collateral) arteries may open up that bypass the block and keep the tissue beyond the block supplied with blood.

Congestive heart failure. A condition resulting from weakness of the heart muscle, which loses its pumping ability. Fluid backs up in the lungs, and may also accumulate in the legs.

Coronary arteries. The arteries supplying the heart muscle with blood—hence, coronary artery disease and coronary heart disease. *Coronary* refers to the heart.

CT (CAT) scan. A computerized X-ray examination.

Diastole. The interval between heartbeats, when the heart is relaxed.

Diastolic blood pressure. The blood pressure trough occurring while the heart is relaxed between beats. It is thus the lower of the two numbers used to describe blood pressure.

Diuretics. Drugs that act on the kidneys to make them excrete more salt and water. They also tend to lower blood pressure.

Echocardiogram. An ultrasound scan of the heart, which can show the movements of the heart valves and the thickness of the muscle.

Edema. Accumulation of fluid, typically in the legs and ankles, which may result from heart failure or as a side effect of some calcium-channel blockers.

Electrocardiogram (ECG or EKG). A tracing of the electrical action of the heart made by attaching recording electrodes to the chest and limbs.

Endothelium. The thin and delicate layer of cells lining the inner walls of blood vessels. Endothelial cells are also chemical factories that produce a variety of substances that can make the vessels both constrict and dilate.

Epinephrine. A hormone released by the adrenal glands that stimulates the heart and dilates the arteries. It is also known as adrenaline.

Free radicals. Unstable chemicals formed in the body, often as products of oxygen metabolism (oxidation). They can cause all sorts of damage to the cells of the body, leading to both vascular disease and cancer. They are mopped up by antioxidants.

Hormone. A chemical messenger; a substance that is formed in one part of the body and circulates in the blood to produce its effects in another part.

Hyperaldosteronism. A condition resulting from an excessive secretion of aldosterone, from either a tumor or other causes.

Hyperkalemia. Too much potassium in the blood.

Hypertension. High blood pressure.

Hypokalemia. Too little potassium in the blood.

Hypotension. Low blood pressure.

Labile hypertension. A term sometimes used to describe very variable blood pressure.

Lipid. A blanket term used to describe the different types of cholesterol (LDL, HDL, and VLDL) and fat (triglycerides) in the blood.

mm Hg (millimeters of mercury). The unit of measurement of blood pressure; the height to which the pressure will push a column of mercury.

Palpitation. A sensation of pounding in the chest resulting from an awareness of the pumping of the heart.

Peripheral resistance. The resistance offered by the blood vessels to the flow of blood. When the vessels are constricted, the resistance is increased, and when they are dilated, it is reduced.

Pheochromocytoma. A tumor of the adrenal gland that secretes hormones (catecholamines) that raise the blood pressure.

Placebo. A Latin word meaning "I will please." Used to describe treatment that has no specific physiological or chemical effect, but that may produce both subjective and objective benefits.

Platelet. The smallest of the circulating blood cells. The chief function of platelets is to form plugs on damaged areas of the linings of the blood vessels and to initiate blood clots.

Postural hypotension. A decrease in blood pressure that occurs on standing.

Potassium. A mineral found in the cells of the body and occurring in several foods.

Preeclampsia. A combination of high blood pressure, ankle swelling, and protein in the urine that may occur during the last three months of pregnancy. Also known as toxemia of pregnancy.

Prostaglandins. A family of chemicals made in the body that have a variety of actions relating to blood pressure regulation and blood clotting. Aspirin and related drugs block their synthesis.

Renin. A hormone secreted by the kidney that raises blood pressure by leading to the formation of angiotensin.

Salt. A chemical composed of a combination of sodium and chloride.

Sodium. The mineral that is one of the two constituents of common salt.

Sphygmomanometer. The device used to measure blood pressure.

Stroke. A sudden loss of function of part of the brain as a result of the interruption of its blood supply by a blocked artery (cerebral thrombosis) or by a burst artery (cerebral hemorrhage).

Sympathetic nervous system. One branch of the autonomic nervous system that regulates the heart and blood vessels by releasing catecholamines (epinephrine and norepinephrine), which stimulate the heart and raise the blood pressure.

Systolic blood pressure. The peak blood pressure, which occurs when the heart pumps blood into the arteries. It is thus the higher of the two numbers used to describe blood pressure.

Transient ischemic attack (TIA). A transient stroke where the symptoms last for less than 24 hours, usually caused by a piece of atherosclerotic plaque breaking off and plugging a small artery in the brain. It subsequently dissolves, and blood flow is restored.

Uremia. The accumulation of waste products in the blood that occurs when the kidneys start to fail.

Vascular. Refers to blood vessels.

Vasoconstrictor. A drug or hormone that causes constriction of the blood vessels.

Vasodilator. A drug or hormone that causes dilation of the blood vessels.

Vitamin. Chemicals produced by plants or animals that are required in our diets in very small amounts to maintain normal health and development.

INDEX

abdomen, fat deposited in, 93–94
abdominal aorta, 41
abdominal ultrasound, 179
ACE (angiotensin converting enzyme) inhibitors, 81, 125, 127–28, 258–59, 263
  captopril, 151, 178–79
  list of, 259
  pregnancy and, 149, 151
  racial differences and, 162
  side effects of, 258–59
acupuncture, 236, 308–9
adolescents, obesity in, 92
adrenal glands, 32, 117, 118
  tumors of, 34–35, 165–67, 173, 181
adrenaline (epinephrine), 31, 117, 118, 166–67
adrenergic receptors, 31
Advanced Care Cholesterol Test, 49
Advil, 294–95
Africa, 65
age, aging, 36
  blood lipids and, 142
  blood pressure and, 116, 140–41, 154–55
  exercise and, 101, 240
  salt sensitivity and, 62
  white-coat hypertension and, 134
  see also elderly
age-related hypertension, see systolic hypertension
Agriculture Department, U.S. (USDA), 205–6

Food Guide Pyramid of, 197–200, 199, 202–4
"Alarm Clocks Can Kill You. Have a Smoke" (Whelan), 103
alcohol, 67, 84, 102, 106–8
  heart disease and, 83, 106, 107–8
  hypertension and, 61, 106, 107, 150
  lipids and, 46, 48
aldosterone, 32, 166, 171
aldosteronomas, 165–66, 181
alpha blockers, 31, 256–57
alpha receptors, 31, 256, 257
alpha-tocopherol (vitamin E), 21, 74, 278–83, 287, 306
alternative medicine, 278, 304–9
American Heart Association (AHA), 42, 52, 61, 142
  diet recommended by, 73, 74, 78, 84, 194, 197–98, 198, 201, 204, 213
American Indians, obesity and, 89
Americans with Disabilities Act, 34
amino acids, 79, 85, 285–86
amphetamine, 226, 227
aneurysm, 32
anger, 36, 119
angina pectoris, 33, 41, 124–26, 140
  treatment of, 124–26, 256, 281
angioplasty, 125–26, 165
angiotensin I, 31–32, 258
angiotensin II, 32, 258
angiotensin blocking agents, 259

ABOUT THE AUTHOR

Thomas Pickering is Professor of Medicine and Associate Director of the Hypertension Center at the New York Hospital–Cornell Medical Center in New York. Born in England and educated at Cambridge Middlesex Hospital in London, and at Oxford, Dr. Pickering is both an M.D. and a Ph.D. (D.Phil.). He is on the editorial board of twelve medical journals, and is a frequent lecturer at national and international medical meetings on hypertension, as well as making frequent appearances on network television. Honors include the British Heart Foundation's Young Investigator Award, several research grants from the National Institutes of Health, and invited lectureships. He is a former president of the Academy of Behavioral Medicine Research, and is secretary of the American Society of Hypertension. He lives in New York City and in Dover, New York.